MW01688568

100% YOU FORMULA

Discover your very own Divine Human Blueprint and the skill to access more energy, vitality and joy with Quantum Energy!

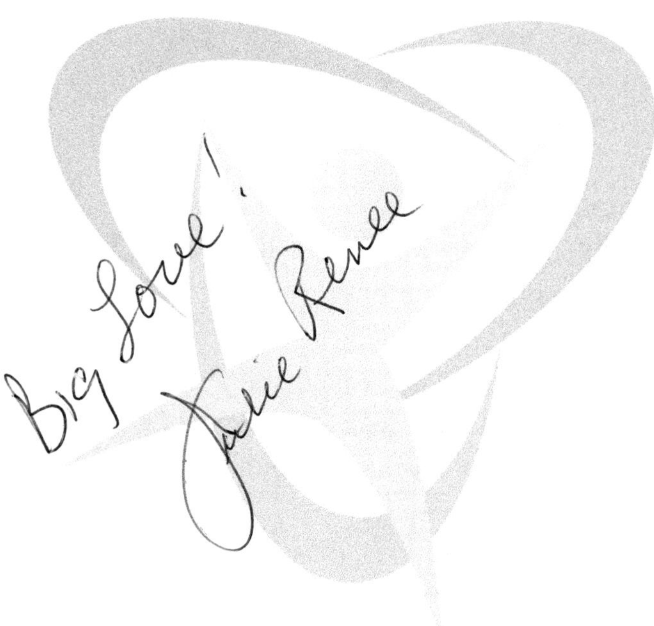

Julie Renee

100% You Formula
by Julie Renee

Copyright ©2013 Gable-Kennedy Publications All Rights Reserved.

Printed in the U.S.A.

ISBN-13: 978-0-9970044-0-3

Visit Julie Renee on the World Wide Web
http://www.julierenee.com
Julie Renee Radio

Terms of Use – Disclaimer
No part of this book may be reproduced or transmitted in any form or by any means, electronic or mechanical, including photocopying, recording or by any information storage and retrieval system without written permission of the publisher, except for the inclusion of brief quotations in a review.

Warning – Disclaimer
The purpose of this book is to educate and entertain. The author and/or publisher does not guarantee that anyone following the techniques, suggestions, tips, ideas or strategies will become successful. The author and/or publisher shall have neither liability nor responsibility to anyone with respect to any loss or damage caused, or alleged to be caused, directly by the information in this book.

Endorsement – Disclaimer
Reference herein to any specific commercial products, process, or service by trade name, trademark, manufacturer, or otherwise, in no manner endorses or sponsors the products, processes or offerings.

Also by JulieRenee

Books

- **Your Divine Human Blueprint**
- **Quantum Healing Secrets**
- **Awakening the Healthy Human**
- **Balance Your Life Now**
- **Breaking Through**

Programs

- **Quantum Mindset Mastery**
- **Quantum Mind—the Four Pillars of Human Mastery**
- **Quantum Healing Secrets**
- **Quantum Success Activations**
- **Accelerate Wealth 21 Day Transformation**
- **Beautiful from the Inside Out—60-Day Makeover**
- **The Sound of Truth: Vedic Mantras**
- **Illumination: The New Rosary**
- **The Definitive Guide Meditation Series**
- **Essence**
- **100% Energy**
- **100% Full Body Ownership**
- **100% Clear**
- **Discovery**
- **Freedom from Spiritual Parasites and Pasts**
- **Julie Renee's Year of Miracles**
- **Diamond Quantum Ambassador Training**

Music

- Gratitude: India classical influence harp and vocals
- Pleasures: Celtic harp and vocals
- The Message: Rumi Love Poetry
- Illumination: Harp

Videos

- Quantum Activations Free Series
- Regeneration: Healing the Glands of the Brain
- Birth Massage Training Video

All are available online, and you may order by visiting http://JulieRenee.com/programs

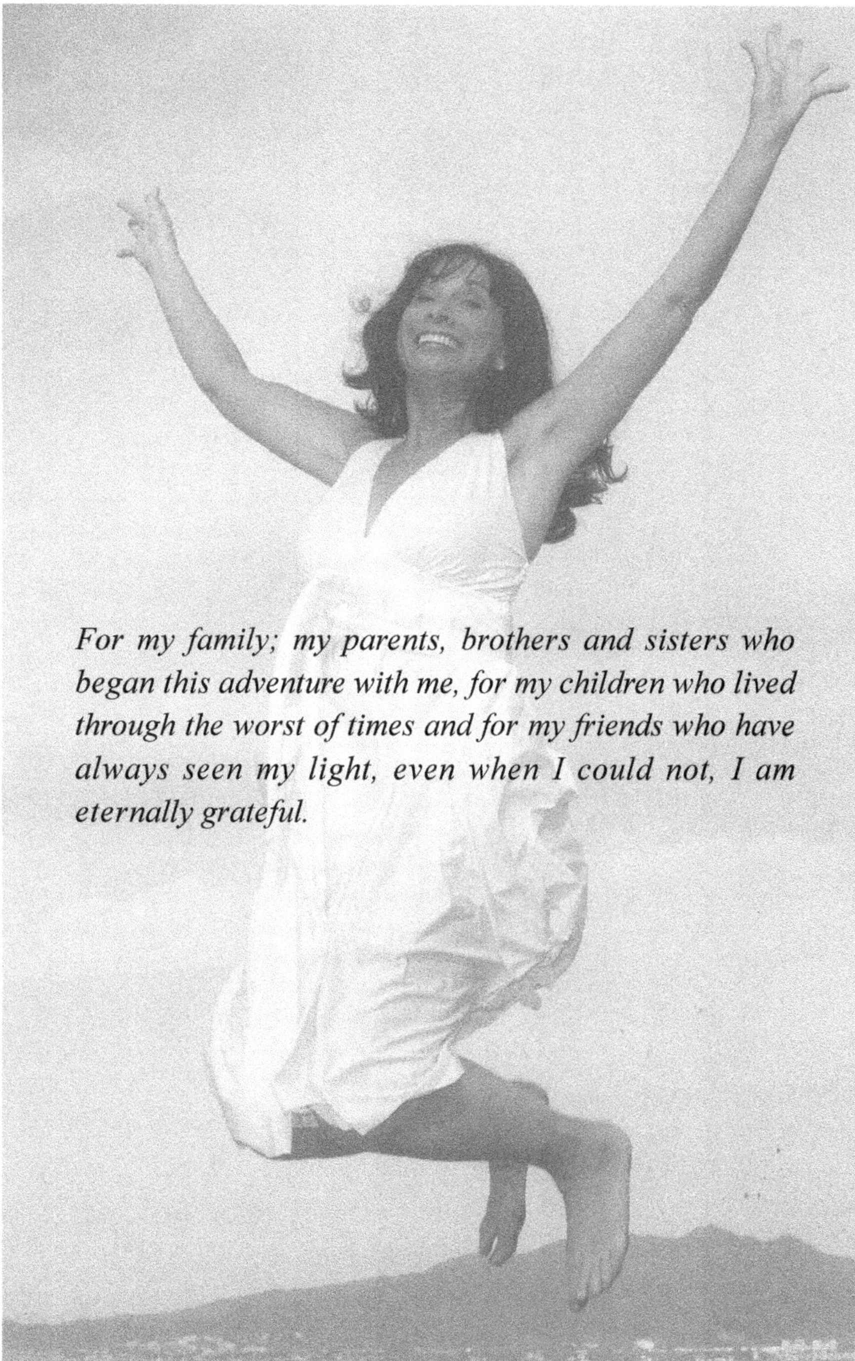

For my family; my parents, brothers and sisters who began this adventure with me, for my children who lived through the worst of times and for my friends who have always seen my light, even when I could not, I am eternally grateful.

TABLE OF CONTENTS

PREFACE

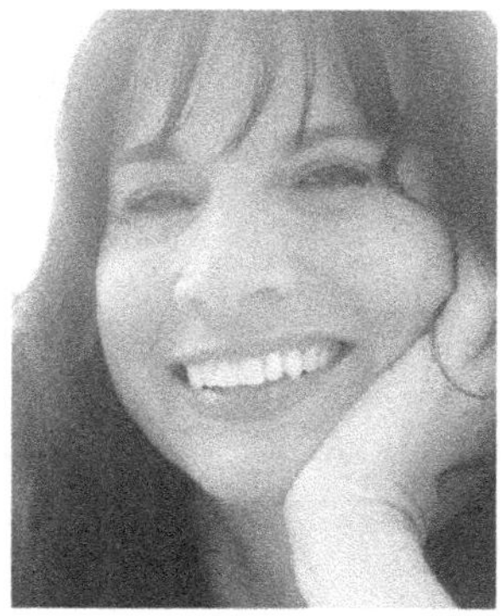

Welcome! My name is Julie Renee and I want to take you on a journey to witness what I believe is the biggest opportunity in vitality, health, wealth, love and receiving in a grand way since the human race first stepped onto planet earth.

That's a big, fat, bold claim and I WANT you to be skeptical. Having said that, I can promise you that when you spend a few minutes with this book and the companion videos, you'll agree with me or at least experience a profound discovery about yourself.

If you don't know who I am or have never heard of me before, there's a short chapter ahead and a video you can watch to "meet" me and find out how I can help you move from wherever you are in your life and success limits to becoming 100% healthy, wealthy, and in love with your life! I'll help you finally put yourself first and foremost and get the vibrant body and lifestyle that has always been part of you and that you so deserve!

Here's a short video: **http://100YouBook.com.**

I've spent nearly twenty-two years helping people just like you overcome health issues and restore their health in phenomenal ways. My clients have included a top-level NASA astronaut, a Google VP, Pentagon officials and a United Nations Ambassador, Hollywood actors and even members of the liturgical profession. My students include members from the sciences, physics, psychiatry, internal medicine, theology, surgeons, holistic health practitioners and professional people from all walks of life, who are excited to learn the secrets I'm about to share with you in this book. I'm about to give you the number one secret for accessing the Divine Human Blueprint—the "magic button"—truly, the "silver bullet" to living a 100% healthy life. By applying these very basic principles, you can dramatically change your life and multiply your healthy, happy years.

Think about it like this: If I could put you in a time machine where you could capture the age of your best health, and keep all the knowledge and wisdom you have today, how would that change your life right now?

If you could have the youthful body you once had and gain the know-how and skill to keep your body that way, while never losing the wisdom and learned intelligence you've acquired from your years of life doing research and development, what would the possibilities for contribution, love, and even wealth acceleration hold for you?

With the content of this book and the videos I've created for you, you can be living 100% with all the benefits of vitality, focus, clarity, and increased energy you desire for the rest of your long life. You could be back playing your best game in a matter of a few short months!

If you have been seeking and searching for years for the SECRET that can literally turn around your life, your intimate relationships, your vitality, and your organic power, you've found it. If you have been searching for how to work more efficiently with precision and motivation than you ever have before (**while you** enhance your quantum field in order to receive more wealth), you've found it.

I discovered how to turn everything in my life around recently when I faced the prospect of choosing to live in suffering, with extreme pain and dysfunction—or embrace the idea of letting go. You see, when I was a child, I survived the underground atomic bomb testing in the Nevada desert. Additionally, our family loved to travel. Mom and Dad would load all five kids in a station wagon with a big Avion trailer in tow. Without knowing it, somehow I got enough toxic exposure to turn my youthful health into a fight for my life at age twenty-four. I was pregnant with baby number three. In short order, I had seventeen surgeries, multiple cancers, and five Near-Death experiences in which I died twice. I spent a year in a wheelchair and was told I would never walk without pain and that I would need to rely on canes.

Then, seven short years ago, a pivotal moment occurred. I made out my will, and for the first time, I instructed my oldest daughter to not resuscitate me if one more "bad" thing happened to me. I thought she needed to let me go, but her response made me think twice about everything: "Mom, I don't want your money. I want you."

I mulled her words over for a week, when it came to me: I was promised the Garden of Eden. I was not meant to live in pain and suffering; I was meant to experience great joy, ecstasy and pleasure in this life.

I went to my garden and declared: **"God take me or make me well."**

And that's when the "downloads" for the 100% Healthy Divine Human Blueprint began pouring in. I had opened Heaven's doorway, I could not only see how poor health affected others and myself, but I could also see how the Blueprint could restore each of us to a younger healthier phase.

When I decided to share this precious, hard-earned knowledge and wisdom with you, it gave me tremendous joy. My life and all the extreme challenges I endured somehow made perfect sense. One of my favorite truths to share is: *"You are always exactly where you need to be, no matter how things may seem to appear."*

This is amazing, because right now you are here with me. We are making a journey together. You are not alone. I am here with you now, because of you. You are my passion and purpose.

Enjoy this book and the videos.

—Julie Renee

Here's what people are saying about the 100% You Formula *and working with Julie Renee's system*

"Julie Renee has written an absolutely fascinating book on 'transformational healing.' Her miraculous and indomitable spirit is everywhere in the book. And yet, the book is about more than healing or 'energy.' The reader comes away with a deep and transforming understanding of the Divine Human Blueprint for health, personal wholeness and success. She offers the reader a fresh look at how to find access to, and become, a 'super star' in your own life and community. I have personally worked with Julie Renee and have been a part of her fabulous workshops. This book captures so much of the magic of those moments. It is not only well-written and inspiring, but it touches the deep places in your soul that have been crying out for a way to escape the mundane and all those limiting circumstances in your life, so that you can fly with the deep aspirations of your soul and heart. The book is more than a 'good read.' It is a doorway and an opportunity to redesign your life in ways that begin on the physical level but quickly affect all the ways you energetically show up in life. If you want to play the game of life at 100% capacity in many ways and levels, this is the book to buy."

Gary D. Salyer, Ph.D., Safe to Love Again Workshop

"Julie Renee is the most extraordinary healer alive today. And I say to everyone, run to Julie Renee versus walk—Run!"

Berny Dorhman Founder of CEO Space

"Clients have been generating with effortless ease. I seem to possess magical abilities. My phone is ringing. I'm receiving checks and commissions in the mail. Money is multiplying literally overnight. I'm so excited. I literally find checks in the mail. I get calls from clients who want to use my services and are ready now. I'm noticing grace and ease throughout my life. I am receiving bigger acknowledgements on stages and invitations to speak have multiplied. One just came in from New Zealand.

Additionally, a cruise just got offered to me. Life is very good. I give credit to Julie Renee for developing this course, for helping me get grounded in my life. Thank you, Julie Renee."

Jill Lublin Author of the *New York Times* Best Seller,
Guerrilla Publicity and Publicity Crash Course

"Julie Renee is a global thought leader in the field of quantum level healing. What makes her work so extraordinary is that her system is so masterful and her results are so rapid. You are in for a luscious treat when you open yourself to the tremendous healing of her work. She is indeed a precious treasure."

Eli Davidson,
Speaker, Coach and Author of *Funky to Fabulous*

"I have been working on Julie Renee's program. The process I have been going through day by day is nothing short of a miracle. Things are really starting to open up. I am getting real clarity and connections to people I have never spoken with before. There is an energy

in the air around me that says whatever it is I am doing, I am doing the right thing. Thank you, Julie Renee"

Jacquliene Wales,
Author of *The Fearless Factor* and *When the Crow Sings*

"Before working with Julie Renee I was feeling tired, burnt out, and older than my years. After working with Julie Renee's program I had the same energy level I remember having when I was fourteen years old! Julie has been able to clear and heal emotional and physical patterns that no other practitioner has ever been able to heal. I highly recommend working with Julie if you struggle with fatigue and chronic health issues that are holding you back from experiencing incredible health."

Cary Peters, Health and Business Coach
Owner, Holistic MBA

"My 12-year speaking business was booming until I hit a dry spell this past year. Despite many marketing campaigns, I was struggling to get booked and my attitude and mindset weren't good. I connected with Julie Renee and she was able to activate my healthy brain and thoughts. Within 5 days of the session, I booked 2 events and I know there are many more to come!"

Karen Phelps Speaker and Trainer, MLM

"Just when you think you have heard it all, you haven't. Not until you read and experience Julie Renee. Her unique and powerful formula for designing your life, for your greatest expression, is in your hands. What a gift! Julie Renee is a leading edge teacher connecting with thought and business leaders who are ready to finally say YES!"

Rae Zander,
Host of the Unity.fm radio show "Everyday Attraction"

Live every day as if it were your first, in awe and wonder.
Live every day as if it were your last,
in gratitude and appreciation

100% YOU!

The Ultimate 5-Step Restart Formula to Help You Become Healthy, Happy, and in Love with Your Life NOW!

Have you ever imagined yourself receiving an award on stage? Perhaps you've imagined a Nobel Peace Prize, an International Leadership Award, or possibly winning a cross-fit competition or dance competition. Have you ever imagined improving your health and vitality so much that your future holds many more additional years than your elders? What if you could not only overcome illness, injury, and suffering, but you could live at 100%? Imagine every part of your body working at 100%, your relationships working at 100%, and your wealth being at 100%.

What if you could use this vitality, focused energy, and organic power to speak to and to serve millions of people? What if you could not only have lots of great ideas, but you could have the clarity, focus and momentum to implement? Imagine you getting your vision out in the world with grace and ease. Imagine being recognized for your talents, accomplishments and expertise. Imagine the impact and influence you could wield with your 100% life. Finally, you'd have the life you so deserve.

If this describes you, I know what you are craving, what you are about, and where you would like to go. What's more? I also know what's standing in your way.

My guess is you have a burning desire to contribute to make a difference, **and** to have the energy, vitality and focus to fulfill your vision of a big life of contribution. You want to have—you've got to have—100% YOU present with focus, clarity, strength and your best energy in order to help people.

You're an entrepreneur or small business owner; you're a mother or father, a professional, or a creative type. And most likely, you've been operating and creating your vision from a much lower function of vitality than the 100% mark. Until you picked up this book, it may never have dawned on you that you could create life from 100%. I don't mean to undervalue the life you have already created. It may be enjoyable and it may be workable, and maybe it's even rewarding. But at the end of the day, you are still in a body that is not functioning at 100%. And when all is said and done, you are breaking down, aging in a degenerative pattern and you haven't discovered the secrets for regeneration.

You know there's more to life. You realize with each passing day your time to impact the world appears to be finite. It's a vicious cycle; if you had more energy or slept better, or if you could just focus or get momentum back, you might have what you need to see your legacy, your mission, manifest in the world. You realize that if you simply stay on the track you are on now, that time will run out, you may lose your opportunity to fulfill your vision, or you may already have settled into a half-life, convinced that 'it's just the way it is" or "that's just how life works." Group mind hypnosis—believing that things are the way they are because that's the way everyone else thinks they are—and a short degenerative life cycle (living less than 150 years) may be the only reality you have ever known.

You also sense something else is possible. Somewhere inside you a dim memory of your own Divine Human Blueprint still eggs you on. It is the thing we call hope, what inspires the envisioning and sends a rippling echo from deep within you: *"I always knew living fully, or 100%—healthy, happy and in love with my life—was possible."*

You want to stop living a half-life and start living at 100% every day. You want to trade in your fuzzy brain, exhaustion, and sleeplessness for brilliance, momentum, and deep, fulfilling rest so you can live fully self-expressed. You want your 100% life and lifestyle NOW so you can experience the preciousness and value of your life well-lived. You want and need to proactively access all of your potential, and open up to new knowledge, vitality and possibilities for freedom, control and independence!

This book is about you, the ambitious, powerful leader who refuses to play small but who is sometimes taken out of the game by exhaustion and fuzzy brain. I want for you to become the 100% YOU SUPER STAR in your life and community so you can live your best life and put yourself first and foremost. And then you'll have all you need to act upon your personal mission and fulfill your dreams, and create your legacy to the fullest.

Whether you are physically or financially in pretty good shape, have a few challenges, or are really struggling, this book is about you getting back to freedom. There are many options for you to improve your health, wealth, vitality and energy in the world today. The choices are endless, and if you are a beginner or have tried lots of ineffective options, selecting your perfect path may seem daunting. Fortunately, once you access your personal Divine Human Blueprint, great internal movement can occur. The shifts in your health and wealth can quickly result because we will be working with your own internal system, saving you years of time, research, money and effort.

The following pages are designed to turn your inner awareness and already good life into a 100% reality that gives you incredible access, authority, and momentum to help you create a wealthy lifestyle effortlessly. And you want to know the best part? Your quantum field will become your wealth magnet, effortlessly.

Ask yourself, What is my motivation and reason for doing what I do?

Are you committed to yourself in this purpose? So often, Entrepreneurs don't include themselves in their mission and vision. They leave themselves last, out of getting all the goodies and upgrades before their clients and students do. Understand that you cannot give what you do not have. I studied healing with sound in India. Sanskrit is the language of truth, where what you speak is the sound of what you are talking about. English is 12% true and is a descriptive language. And like our culture and behaviors, very few individuals lead from their essence, resonating with their truth (experience of life). When you put yourself, your health, your home, your personal relationships, and your bank account before what you give to others, you become the example and the new standard of truth in business.

YOUR OPPORTUNITY

Have you ever stopped to realize that being 100% is possible?

I'm going to go out on a limb now. I have a feeling I also know *exactly why* you're struggling to succeed at BEING 100%. I know why you have not been "healed" or "cured" or "fixed." I know why your intent has not paralleled your efforts

First and most importantly, know this: The problem is not *you*.

Both the "diagnosis" and "cure" for your living 100% in health, vitality, wealth, and good relationships can be summarized in one simple, yet seemingly elusive, concept.

Are you ready?

The concept is **Your Divine Human Blueprint**.

That's it. You have a Divine Human Blueprint, which holds the encoding for your 100% healthy, happy life. My hunch is that what you are currently lacking is access to the ancient knowledge that was wired into you—and all humans—from the beginning of humankind. No matter how awesome your medical and alternative practitioners are, no matter how awesome your wellness program is, or even how amazing you are, or how much heart you bring with you into everything you do, if you aren't accessing the design you are created from, well, it just doesn't matter. You'll want to acquire a significant knowledge of your own Divine Human Blueprint, or align with a group of people who understand the Divine Human Blueprint and care about you and your full return to 100%.

In this book, I'm going to do my very best to inspire you and give you the tools you need to get started on accessing your magnificent design. Ultimately, I want you to be able to restore and regenerate whatever troubles you, activate your best life, and live your life so fully expressed that you create a life you never dreamed was even possible.

I also want to give you a huge gift. I want to help you get focused, clear, and full of energy. I want you to be able to touch into your Divine Human Blueprint and activate your best health. As a start, I'd like to gift you with my 100% You mastery courses: the first course is Dynamism—how to access all of your energy resources from your Divine Human Blueprint.

The second course is The Law of Generosity: This course includes a guided meditation to magnetize wealth to you rapidly. You'll discover important new awareness and access to your "plan" using the 100% You mastery courses. Gorgeous guided imagery and the sound of melodious harp strings help to make the process of acquiring new awareness and health simple and effortless.

Are you intrigued?

I know I am promising you the moon, so to speak, and I know I'm going to have to prove the authenticity and power of the Divine Human Blueprint to you. Don't worry. I've helped a number of high profile clients—from a top-level NASA astronaut, to a Stanford scientist, a Google executive, Pentagon officials, a United Nations Ambassador, Hollywood actresses, three *New York Times* bestselling authors, and professionals from sciences such as physics, psychiatry, internal medicine, theology, surgery, holistic health practitioners, and professional people, as well as a whole lot of people just like you.

I'd like to share the same systematized health activations I did with these high level thought leaders with you because these same techniques will help you, too.

I'd also like to share with you the five elements of your Divine Human Blueprint so that you can shift from a Band-Aid fix for your life, in which you are just getting by while still trying to figure out how to do better, to a 100% restoration, in which health is your natural state of being and all manner of goodness flows to you—simply, easily and effectively.

Open your eyes every day. As the Sufi poet said, "My God, when I open my eyes and really see what you have given me, my heart is overflowing and my eyes are filled with tears."

MY STORY

Out of the darkness and into the Light

It all began at North Memorial Hospital in Robbinsdale, Minnesota. I grew up with two brothers and two sisters in a middle class family in the suburbs. I can't say that, as a child, I ever question my own mortality. Oh, just like you, I had the usual childhood catchable stuff, such as measles, mumps, chicken pox, and an occasional cold, but for the most part, I was healthy. I did have one unique condition, though; I "chose" not to speak. I probably would have been diagnosed as autistic had I been born today, but that was another time.

Oddly, when I was age three, my pediatrician told my mother that if they removed my tonsils and adenoids, I would speak. Well, that didn't work. But I figured if I didn't start making sounds they **would** take more out. So, though not intelligible, I made sounds resembling words till I got into school. Once in school, I learned how to hear and replicate sounds and words, and after two years of speech therapy, I had the best pronunciation of words in my elementary school. Actually, that whole experience has been an amazing blessing. I learned I could master anything with practice, even things that weren't natural to me. The second blessing was that I became an incredible listener. I went on to study voice as a classical vocalist and have sung in nineteen languages. Many of those I replicated so well native speakers assumed I spoke their language.

When I was about twelve, my family went on vacation to the Nevada desert. We were all great travelers and loved the adventure. By this time, I had eight years of camping under my belt. I got lucky and got to sleep in a pup tent with my big brother.

What we didn't pay attention to on our holiday was that the U.S. government was doing underground bomb testing near our adventure. Somehow, I, like many others who are referred to as "down winders," got a dose of radiation that would change my future permanently.

Why I got the worst of things we'll probably never know. But at age twenty-three on December 2, 1980, I learned that I had terminal cancer. Wow! What a shocker! Not to mention I was four months pregnant with baby number three. Imagine being in a loveless marriage, a baby on the way, and no apparent way back to health.

Though I didn't have the Divine Human Blueprint information back then that I have now, my faith was unshakable. I believed God personally loved me and would help me out of this certain death.

The sequence of major events that year evolved like this: pregnancy, in four months-major surgery, at six months- surgery, at nine months-delivery of an eight-pound baby boy (my own weight was 104 pounds), only weeks after birth-major surgery, six months after birth-radiation therapy, multiple hospitalizations, two minor surgeries, weakness, frailty, fainting away, and dying alone. My body collapsed, but I pushed my spirit back into it and reanimated my body, after which I suffered separation, divorce, and a break down. Oo la la! I do hope you haven't lived a year like that. I have found that no matter what our challenges are, they are all big to us, because they are our personal challenges.

Now that was the year I will always remember for what I discovered:

- We are radiant
- We are beings of light
- Life is not over unless we say it is
- Faith, which is part of perception, can help you overcome many difficulties

I hadn't a clue yet how everything worked. Thank God for faith, hope, and love, which carried me till I could comprehend and translate the intricate workings of the Divine Human Blueprint and begin the wise elder journey of implementing my own health activations for restoring my health where no other options were possible.

When all was said and done, I had seventeen surgeries, two cancers, ten years of radiation treatment, five Near-Death experiences, a year in a wheel chair, two major brain injuries, and a whole heck of a lot of PAIN.

You might be wondering how I went through all that, and more importantly, how I got to be the healthy, happy woman I am today.

I learned how to be a receiver, and I learned how to let the good in.

Remember, I told you I had become a really good listener? Well, that isn't the half of it. While working as a graphic artist for the police department in downtown Minneapolis at the age of twenty-six, my body would receive WCCO radio. Yes, out of my chest, my office mates heard the announcers covering the news. It's funny, but I will never forget the words, "...and it's Harmon Killebrew at bat! He's hit a home run!"

Well, with that kind of receivership, you can probably imagine the challenges I have had with technology and the blessings I have had in being a clear space for connection and reception to the Divine.

One day a few years ago, I'd reached my end emotionally. Maybe on some level you've had a moment like that. It's not depression; it's a firm resolve that things are going to change. My perception shifted. I was no longer interested in survival; I was interested in the "promise of the Garden of Eden" life. I wanted a life without pain. Some people call it thriving, but it was more than that; I was going to return to 100% or I wanted out of this pain-wracked body.

Remember these two ideas: 'resolve' and a 'perception shift' because they are important to you if you are going to make a big change in your life.

I went to my garden with a firm resolve. I demanded that God either take me or make me well. If you are a follower of the Buddha, you will know that is how Buddha became enlightened. It was thought that the rich, such as beings like Buddha, who was a prince, could not reach enlightenment unless they threw away their wealth and became poor Sadhus. With a firm resolve, Buddha sat under a Bodhi tree for forty days. However long it took, he would stay in meditation till he reached enlightenment.

And so he did.

I went to my little prayer garden every day where I sat in prayer, meditated, and chanted songs of devotion. However, as I did, I fell in love with the Divine. I moved away from remembering pain and began to dream of oneness and freedom. And I began to see even on that first day, that my Divine Human Blueprint was restoring itself. I watched a master stem cell rise from an abysmal low function to attain functional perfection. When it reached the state of oneness, it burst open into a pulsing blue spheroid shape. As I witnessed this profound event, I burst into tears. I felt I was looking into the face of God, intense and beautiful.

I have rarely seen the actual transformation since, yet it is subtle and easy. You don't need to be a visionary or be a big receptor to experience the stem cells in your body returning to perfection or see them teaching the surrounding cells how to do the same. You, too, with the correct perception and resolve, can access your system of regeneration that has always been yours to access.

I had already been a healer. From the beginning, I was a massage therapist for people in recovery from addiction and trauma. After a few years, I specialized in therapeutic and sports injury, which naturally lead to auto accident recovery. That opened the door to medical massage. At this point, I possessed a great deal of skill as a master masseur, favored by the local ob/gyn and midwife community. I was more than busy, assisting women with high risk pregnancies as well as assisting with their deliveries and performing infant massage after the births.

During those years, I was certified in more than a dozen modalities and studied herbal medicine, flower essences, and essential oils to compliment the work I was doing with my clients. Eventually, I added homeopathy.

My breakthrough and blessings involved being able to give a special, unique gift of healing to everyone I touched. Women who worked with me stopped having hot flashes, PMS symptoms, and migraines, just from simply having a massage or two. It was exciting to see the miracles, and I continued to improve also. In that first year, I threw the walking cane away. I started running long distances again and was a regular stage dancer with the local Doc Kraft band.

I needed to start charting what I was doing so I could show how I was getting such great results. With my inner eye, I could watch the cellular bodies of my clients improve, and I started mapping out what we were doing that made the shifts happen. All this time, I relied entirely on the body of the person who was receiving the healing to show me where to go next.

During the process, I noticed that my clients' perceptions and mindsets could be deterrents from time to time. A resistant nature, a curse, or even someone's DNA program could get in the way of a full healing.

This forced me to look at the role of perception/mindset in healing. I discovered that "group mind hypnosis" was creating a great deal of the stuck disharmonic challenges in my clients. This means that if someone believes that something cannot be different just because 'it has always been this way,' that perception will deter their healing. Clearing these issues levels the playing field so everyone can get the improvements they want.

From the moment of my first health activation that first day in the garden, my thoughts were about how to help others get out of suffering and pain. Through the years I had helped so many suffering individuals, but without the knowledge of the Divine Human Blueprint there was only so far we could go.

As time passed, I began to develop word-of-mouth fame, but my schedule became overwhelmingly busy. I would often do more than sixty hours of healing each week, and on travel weeks, I would teach in the evenings and do seventy hours of client healing time with no real breaks for meals. I would simply stuff a sandwich in my mouth and keep working.

Eventually, my clients asked me to teach them the methods I used to do—the more complex processes, and an apprentice program was born. This began as a fly-by-the-seat-of-your-pants training, but by the time the fourth weekend rolled around, I was organized and providing both written chapters and training videos for my students to absorb the information. The students were professional people with busy schedules who were excited to learn a new way of improving health.

While my program was foundationally very good, a few important pieces still needed to be filled in. The program morphed into an immersion program so that students could absorb the Divine Human Blueprint in their core. The program shifted from eight weekends and numerous trainings, to five two-day trainings over the course of a year, making it more accessible for professionals, who could incorporate the teachings into their active schedules. Secondly, I created a tighter, more intimate group that could go through the entire year together. With everyone in sync having the same information and with everyone taking their training at the same time, the group became more intimate, allowing lots of time for me to give the trainees my personal attention.

I don't know about you, but I can take a good guess that you are a bit like me: you want to contribute, feel great, and really enjoy the life you have been given. I like watching the Oscar, Academy Award, and Grammy shows on TV. It's exciting to watch actors and musicians being recognized as the best at what they do, a similar excitement for me as when I watch Olympic sporting contests; it's just thrilling.

Can you imagine yourself at the top of your field? Can you imagine playing with all of your cylinders firing? For me, it's not about the fame and fortune; I just want to feel like I've lived my very best life, without regrets, and without feeling like I "woulda, coulda if only I'd had more energy and vitality." That's not how I wanted to look back at my life.

I want to feel like I've made my mark by working consciously and with perseverance, and that I loved and helped a lot of folks in the process. I could do that to a certain extent when I was functioning only halfway, but if I could use the total amount of my energy, focus, and momentum, my positive influence could expand even more, as can yours.

From the deepest fibers of my being, that's what inspires me and reconfirms my commitment to living a life of service to help transform lives, one person at a time, so that each of them may, in turn, create his/her ripple effect to increase the total amount of goodness in the world. Although money and recognition feel nice in the moment, those benefits are mere by-products of what really matters to me on this more profound level.

Here's the address of a short two minute video about my goals and motivations: **http://100YouBook.com.**

Self Care ~ You Choose
Maintaining good energy throughout the day may mean setting a timer to accomplish only part of a task before getting up and stretching or going for a walk. If you treat your body like a slave, it will behave like a slave and you will not send out the signals of a powerhouse, but rather of an indentured servant.

YOUR JUICE

{!!!}

Okay, so what about you? What's your inspiration?

What lights you up? What motivates you? What is your big WHY? What inspires you to live your best, and now your 100% best, every day? What could you do if you knew you had clarity, focus, energy, momentum, and the ability to sustain it? What are the wins you might experience with this kind of life? Who besides you would get a big benefit from your momentum? Whose life would get better because you are now functioning at 100%?

Doesn't it feel great to dream? Getting fully connected to your vision and outcome is an important step. Feel "into it." How does your body feel at 100%? How about your mind? What's your energy like? Can you taste and smell at 100% differently than you do now?

Let's get down to it. If you could have all aspects of your health, vitality, mind and energy—**everything**—working a lot better, what would it feel like? Just for now, let's **not** make a list of what's wrong, but let's take a few minutes to dream. In your journal, write a minimum of ten declarations in response to the statement: "How I feel, now that I am 100%".

In contrast, how would it feel if you knew nothing would ever improve, or that you would never live your life to the fullest, impact the people you love, or serve in a bigger way? Why would that be so bad?

Imagine the frustration of not being able to get your work out in the world, never being acknowledged for your contributions, or maybe never really being with your loved ones the way you could be? Imagine never making a difference—imagine losing more energy and focus as you live a half-life for the rest of your days.

Take time now to write in your journal about how much you have lost by not improving the areas of challenge you currently struggle with. Approach this task as you would an essay. No one but you will see it, so be honest with yourself and explore what it is costing you to not have some really big breakthroughs.

Be in the daily practice of honing and refining your vision for your life and happiness.

LIFE IS SHORT

I have a confession to make. You know when I found out I had cancer, I already knew it, and if I had not been pregnant I might have just given up: I was trapped in an unhappy marriage because I did not believe in divorce and was weak and tired all the time.

The first time I collapsed on the floor, I weighed ninety-six pounds. I left my body and died. I saw my life flash before me, and what I saw very clearly was a life unfulfilled: I hadn't raised my kids, accomplished my mission in the church, or helped enough mothers and babies. I was clearly not done. Yet my body, to the contrary, was saying very loudly, "End game!" My doctor, kindly, had not told me, but had noted on my chart that the end was near. I had perhaps a week or two at the most.

At the age of twenty-four, I said, "NO! Life cannot be over. No!" I began to recount my reasons for why I must live. I have to tell you, for many years, the saying that "life is short" served me; I lived every day as if it might be my last. Knowing that time is precious has become ingrained in me now. You must live to the fullest each and every moment.

I have a big mission. I have a huge life to live, one that requires me to be fully healthy, wealthy, and in love with life every moment.

Although there are many mysteries in life, I committed to living a 100% healthy life during every precious moment I spend in this Garden of Eden.

I have to admit my life, at least the first part of it, had been extremely difficult. I spent two-and-a-half years of my life in a hospital, for years I was unable to work, and I suffered unending pain for fifteen years. In spite of all of these challenges, I honestly believe I got the life I needed in order to help you. Therefore, wherever you are in your health, whether mostly healthy or only so-so, my mission is to support you on the road to playing full out again.

I am no longer in pain; I have had no cancer for ten years, and plan to never let my body go down that path again. Each day is a new opportunity to bring more light and love into my life and into yours. This is my mission. This is why I am here.

I am not sharing my story and the details of my former health condition to shock you, put you off, or one-up your story; I have no interest in that. I am transparent with you because by knowing some of my story and what I overcame, you can see that I am an example of what is truly possible.

I still work on myself every day. I am not perfect; being close to death so many times has given me ample material to learn and work on. However, I am so healthy, I am completely unrecognizable from just a few years ago, and I continue on my quest for 100% health. However, by experiencing the great health I now feel, I hope I can massively affect global consciousness on creating wellness and a return to great health for others.

My plan for the planet is that I can encourage earth's population, one person at a time, to use their original Divine Human Blueprint in order to gain a body that was created to live hundreds of years. I imagine reaching millions of individuals in all the countries of the world, and showing everyone a simple and easy way back to health and vitality.

Using my tools and techniques developed from accessing the Original Divine Human Blueprint, healthy families and individuals worldwide will live longer, more productive, and truly happier lives!

That's my legacy. That's what I will leave behind and what I want to gift to you. I also want to create 100% health for myself along the way, as well as a life of financial ease and lots of adventure, so I am showing up 100% for myself every day.

If you are reading this right now, I want you to know that I wrote this for you. These are the perfect words you need to read and integrate into yourself right now. You are my purpose. You are my passion. You are the fuel for my resolve. I choose you.

Bringing your health and vitality to 100% functionality is my mission. You living your life 100% full on is what excites me and gives me the push to go further. My dream for you is that you will step into a fuller expression of yourself and become deeper, richer and more of the person you were meant to be, one who can make a big impact on your world and mine! I want you to have the energy, momentum and vitality to realize your full potential. I want to see you share your blessings in the world, and I KNOW you can do this.

This is your time to live 100%. This is your time to shine!

Start each day getting your energy, mindset and body in its best, most receptive mode. This means scheduling in time for exercise, eating nutritiously, and drinking enough water.

YOUR TIME IS NOW

This moment is the perfect time for you to be 100% healthy again, to really feel great in your body, to be able to connect with the ones you love, and the people who are best suited for your mission's fulfillment. The key to your fulfillment lies in your organic nature. By remembering and accessing your Divine Human Blueprint, your own personal instruction manual, you will be able to open the doors to life as you long for it to be. Human history has preserved your Blueprint perfectly, and as we head more deeply into the astrological age that supports greater human access to Divine information, we are, quite possibly for the first time in thousands of years, aligned with our selves—the nature of our true, authentic being. In this age of equality, human history, and our being able to access the wisdom out of which we were created, is more transparent than it has been for eons! Every day there is a new modality, procedure, or supplement brought into the global marketplace for us to try out and test.

However, every human being in a living body will encounter a point at which he or she needs assistance in order to stay healthy. That is why the utility of a system for accessing the Divine Human Blueprint has become far-reaching and powerful. Every human being will, at some point, need the awareness and implementation of wellness found in the Devine Human Blueprint to live a happy, fulfilling life.

Let's talk about your health now. The rules of health care are changing rapidly, and where you might have first turned to a doctor for diagnosis and treatment, now you might try a few different types of treatment to resolve an issue. It is not a given that you will choose surgery over a nutritional program, or that a pill might be more potent than energy work to resolve fatigue. Western medicine tells us that when adrenals fail, they will never work again. Yet, I am now seeing clients whose adrenals have grown back and are at full function within weeks of a "100% You, Elite One-Day" program that I run. The world is changing, and what's so amazing is that, as it changes, we seek out that which is true, so that which resonates within us is becoming our first choice.

Have you noticed how the medical and healthcare giants are now adding yoga and meditation to their tablets and that they are now suggesting supplements, like melatonin and valerian, for rest?

The ability to access the truth in regards to restoring one's health is shifting rapidly, even when one has no expertise. Every day, I hear someone say, "I always knew that was true, deep inside," or "I always thought that was possible," or "it feels right," or "the hair on my arms is standing up, so I know this is true." I have even heard some people I treat say, "I had a dream, and I saw myself working with you, even before I met you. I knew you could complement the awareness I have," or, "My Guides told me I would meet you."

I am actually being transparent again. This really is happening. I think we, as a people, are ready to hear the truth about how we are designed, and the truth is probably not going to come from a big health conglomerate. I want you to understand that it's not because people in the modern health industry are hiding something from you; they really don't have this knowledge.

To embrace the Divine Human Blueprint means both feeling it and knowing it. The old model of medicine is obsolete and irrelevant. Medical knowledge is important for pieces of the Blueprint, but the medical model only addresses the physical body, and moderately addresses perception. Missing are other vital aspects related to restoring health that are found in the Divine Human Blueprint.

Every day, you have choices as to how you will optimize your energy and vitality. Do you drink a latte or a green drink? Do you go for a hike in nature, do yoga, head for a gym workout, or take a pass on exercise today? What are you thinking about? Are your current thoughts the best way to think about that situation, or could you benefit by improving your thoughts? Do you think there might be some new and more useful thoughts that might help you to step over what used to be a roadblock?

We are in an information age. If you are reading this book, you want to learn, and the very fact that you have gotten this far means that you are a seeker.

What if I told you that within five hours you could have your brain functioning at 100% and that new cells would start growing to replace the old cells, providing a complete restoration of your brain cells within 110 days? Does this information excite you? To bring your health, your wealth, your love, and your lifestyle to 100% functionality for you just takes a little effort, the right tools, and the right kind of training.

When you think about the life you can live if all your systems functioned at 100%, the possibilities for achievement and accomplishment are endless. Think about the loving, happy, energized moments you will share with friends, loved ones, the kids, and your folks.

What's more? This information has always been inside you. You have always had a glimmer of it because it is part of your very nature.

Does it excite you to know that the programs for 100% health, wealth, love, and mission fulfillment are already a part of you? [1] *(1. The results reported are based on kinesiology test results from hundreds of clients.)*

It blows me away. I think about how I suffered, and how free I am now to live a fully self-expressed life! Yahoo! I am so jazzed! And this is possible for you, too.

The cool part about the Divine Human Blueprint is that the changes and improvements you make to your health, love, and money are sustainable. The improvements, when made at the deepest level, don't slip away. From the moment your perceptions are cleared, your first health activations will just keep getting better. [2] *(2. If you have deliberately exposed yourself to toxins and brain-killing chemicals, which is the case with most people on the planet, you must consider how you will live with this toxicity or how you will restore yourself to a healthier state.)*

You have a chance right now to change your life, and in so doing, to add to the lives of everyone you love and care about.

I believe the secrets you'll discover in this short book are the easiest and fastest way back to living full out at your personal best! 100%! As an entrepreneur, small business owner, mother, father, or executive, you can experience the incredible shifts of wellness by activating your own natural Divine Human Blueprint that is already inside you. Of course, it's up to you to take action and implement the easy methods I will be showing you to make these shifts happen.

You must prepare yourself for the journey, because the time is now. Whether your life is only 20% or 50% expressed, it doesn't matter; the process is about restoring and reclaiming yourself. Take advantage of the momentum and the incredible information pouring in right now. Don't wait another moment.

So, how are you going to get started? What's the first step when there is such a massive amount of information in the mainstream about healing?

Clean up your diet. Foods with contaminants affect the natural flow of energy and vibrancy in the body. Limit things like packaged and fried foods. Clean up the air you breathe and the water you drink. Use a technology "blocker" on your computer and cell phone and wear another blocker around your neck or wrist to maintain better signal flow and strength.

100% YOU

Healthy, Happy, Wealthy, Energetic, Focused, and in Love with Your Life

So, how do you combine what you already know about living your 100% lifestyle with the hidden Divine Human Blueprint that exists deep within you? It's not necessarily quick and easy. There is no magic pill that makes everything perfect overnight. The fundamentals, which include tools for restoring cells, improving patterns, and brightening and energizing one's self require steady implementation of a paced system.

If you think of it practically, it took you a lifetime to get to where you are now; it may take some time to reverse problems and move towards your 100% goal. You'll want to continue to improve your healthy lifestyle. Nutrition, exercise, and meditation will be part of your journey. Restoring your physical, spiritual, energetic, and perceptual self is the process by which you can restore integrity to all parts of you.

You're simply using the design you were created from—that all humankind was created from—and restoring your internal knowledge and wisdom. Full functionality is accomplished in five easy steps. As you move through each step, you will move closer to your 100% goal.

I've been building and refining an accessible system for over seven years. I've customized it for hundreds of clients and students, but till now, it had to be delivered one person at a time or in small groups. As I have grown in my understanding of the Divine Human Blueprint, the "way in" has continued to get simpler. The first information I received years ago was in the direction equivalent to the fulfillment of a healing task. Just like brain surgery, I would receive the step-by-step process of how to totally restore the brain using cellular quantum mechanics. I got the downloads in that way because that was the intensity and urgency of my own need back then. As the years have passed, the broad stroke and "easy way in" have revealed a much more direct path in.

Up until now, using technology was not an option. Delivery costs for the 100% health activations made it exclusive for the elite few who had big enough bank accounts. That's not the case anymore. In the past twelve months, it has become a real option to use technology for delivery of your 100% healthy system. Now, it is possible for anyone with enough passion and motivation to successfully master this system.

You don't have to be a doctor, holistic practitioner, or even a healer. You don't have to understand science. You don't have to have a pedigree from a fancy school. I sure don't. You don't need a big background in health or a cadillac insurance policy. You don't need a team of doctors, healers, and trainers to get back to 100%. There are no side effects, no lost work, and there is virtually no risk. There is absolutely nothing stopping you from starting immediately.[3] *(3. If you are currently under a doctor's care for a medical condition, you will want to continue till you have mastered your own health activations. Please remember to do nothing abrupt, nothing severe, meaning we don't sever what you have currently in place; rather, you will gently replace what doesn't work as your health returns.)*

However, before you begin, there is one more thing you have to have in place. As I mentioned before, there is one BIG aspect of the Divine Human Blueprint that will be the cornerstone of your success. It is the one factor you have probably been missing. You will discover that this big factor is the self-administered cure to your exhausted, weak, worn, irritable, and broken self.

You can become so strong in your "100% You lifestyle" that your value to yourself and others will rise immensely. Think about being 100% energized, focused and clear. You will be impacting more lives, and as a result, you could be bringing in twice as much capital as you had previously, and possibly much, much more than that. As a result of becoming clearer and more focused, clients often report experiencing less down time or wasted time, have fewer doctors' bills, and clear up debt issues, and painful relationships dissolve. Can you see how having 100% clarity and focus will help you move into freedom?

So, what is the big factor? The big piece is called *perception.*

What exactly is "perception"? It's what you think (your mindset), combined with how you feel (an emotional sensation). It's your unique interpretation of your experience and the field from which you live your life. Think about this concept. It's one that you are very familiar with but probably have never applied to how it affects you now.

Here is how perceptions were formed:

"In the beginning was the Word and the Word was with God and the Word was God." —Genesis

So, before there was what we call, "spirit," before there was a physical form we call "body," and before there were energy and momentum, there was the WORD. The Word the Bible refers to means "perception." How you experience everything—in other words, the creator God you are as you design—or stubbornly refused to design—your life starts with perception. How happy or irritable you are, whether people like or ignore you all happens in your perception.

Please suspend your information about how the word "perception" is used in current language. When I use this term related to the Divine Human Blueprint, it is both that which causes life to play out in a certain way (your mindset) and your emotions interpreting and directing how life will be.

Perception—Understanding the How's and Why's

- Safety of the body is a key factor in the programs enforced by perception
- Is not tied to the body/brain—in other words, the programs in perception are not wired from body or brain programs
- Connects or disconnects you to life and others
- Informs how you let go, clear, or hold on
- Directs all your abilities
- Can be conscious or unconscious
- Can be swayed by group mind and others
- Is manipulated and altered by family programs
- Improves with affirmations, mantras, and being "convinced"
- Requires no special skill or technique; shifting is effortless

To be 100% functional and healthy requires a shift in your perception of how worthy and deserving you are of functioning in all aspects of your life at 100%. You must truly believe you deserve this. A shift towards the ultimate positive in your life can only truly happen when you align your beliefs with your best interests and, in perception, know this is your truth. It's a bit like the story I told where I "knew" in my heart-of-hearts that God did not mean for me to suffer, and I became **aware** of this truth. I then went to my garden and said, *"God take me or make me well. You promised me the Garden of Eden and I am claiming it now."* Improving perception requires that you wake up to new possibilities for yourself.

In this conversation, we are talking about the mindset, or field, you will create your shifts from.

Every single person on the planet who desires to make a shift up to their 100% life needs shifts in the perception towards supporting their desires. In the system of the Divine Human Blueprint, perception is a critical and vital component; it is truly the foundation of your success. With clear perception, you are unstoppable. You're free. This is why all the big coaches and trainers use mindset techniques to amplify their training techniques. The only piece missing is that they don't go back to the source of the design itself and alter it.

Setting your perception at 100% for your life will change everything. Perception accelerates your field for love, money, and health. It brings resources to you, and makes you magnetic and in charge of your life. It is your formula to win-win-win!

Once your perception is upgraded to 100% You, you can sustain and maintain it for the rest of your days.

Let me give you some examples:

A business coach prone to migraines came to me because she'd had too many down days due to her condition. With a shift of perception, she let go of the perception patterns of people taking advantage of her, and her headaches no longer took root.

How does that work, you may ask?

First, we identified an old perception that allowed the headache. Then we identified a perception that it was actually "her headache" and altered that perception to a new belief that nothing that caused her pain was hers. With this new perception, she could easily separate herself from the migraines, and she found herself feeling good 100% of the time. Without the migraines to hold her back, she landed a coaching position in a rising organization and started to fill her own practice, as well. You can, too.

In another example, an ambitious business, health, and wellness coach that really wanted to make her mark in the world was constantly playing second fiddle to her family and friends. Her perception was that she lived only on the success or struggles of her loved ones. With this perception, she left herself no leverage with others, so no matter what she did, she could not make any headway to get her blessings and wisdom out into the world.

Her path has been one of shifting her perception to include new patterns to function from. "Having the right to take up space," and "everybody loves me and wants me to succeed," are the new perceptions that will get her to the ground she can powerfully create from. This improvement in her perception will drive her success and full expression for years to come.

Here is another example: A corporate speaker had difficulty relating to men. She also suffered from a lack of fun time and quality time with her girlfriends. Her needed perception shifts included the following: "I am 100% lovable and loving," " it is an important part of life to have fun with friends," and "it is vital to my well-being to create a new happy life." Over a few weeks, she began to learn about herself in new ways, having fun, and interacting with both men and women in circumstances in which she felt loved and loving.

Another professional speaker went from having a striving personality to becoming a happy, well-balanced, intelligent woman who started booking many more speeches and having more fun! It's easy. It's a total "game-changer" as everything shifts upward in your life when your perception shifts for the better.

It used to be a trendy New Age thing to perform more affirmations. But just doing affirmations alone rarely shifts perceptions, which is why patterns and failures often returned even if there was a temporary improvement. Shifting perception creates changes that are permanent.

Now that you know how important perception is at its deepest level, you can understand that shifting your unique challenges into your greatest wins is a true and lasting gift. It's your commitment, resolve, and willingness to have a new 100% functional life that fuels your momentum and shifts your perceptions.

What is unique about you? What holds you back from sharing your unique gifts and blessings with the world? Are there elements in your perceptions that prevent you from authentically shining?

Once you have cleared your perceptions, you are on your way. The steps that follow ensure that your concerted efforts to live the life you've always imagined can become a reality. We approach your 100% functional life and program with laser-focused clarity and meaningful leaps into your best-ever sustainable life.

I have always found that slowing down and taking my time will get me to my finish line faster than rushing around and making lots of errors. So, I keep it simple and do a few things, but do them really well. Heartfelt work grows purely from a place of strength.

FIVE STEPS IN THE 100% YOU PROGRAM

Easy Access to the 100% YOU Restart Formula from Your Divine Human Blueprint

Here is the *100% You!* formula: PEMER:

1. **Perception**
2. **Essence**
3. **Matter**
4. **Energy**
5. **Realms**

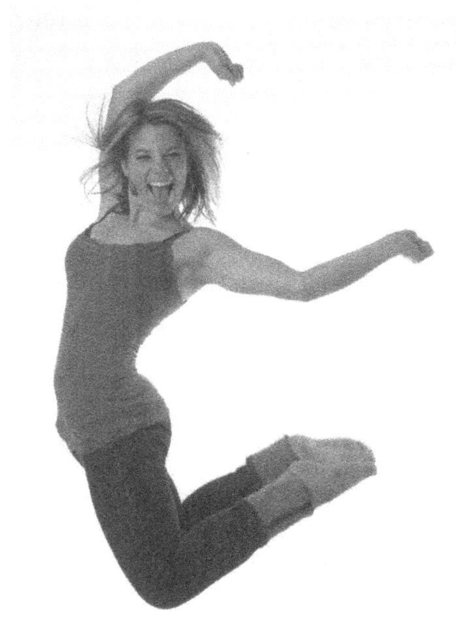

✓ STEP 1: PERCEPTION

To start living your powerful, enduring, 100% healthy, wealthy, happy, and in-love-with-your-life "life," you'll need to clean house in your perceptions. This includes your mindset, emotions, influential group mind and thought forms. You need to open to your biggest, best self to allow the vision of 100% to permeate all parts of you. It's really not that hard.

The key is to first get in touch with your "why." Know what makes you passionate about shifting and virtually altering how you experience life. This is super important. Without your "why," fueling this shift, you will fail. Your "why" drives the momentum through change, good or uncomfortable, but necessary. Your "why" is a key element to succeeding. What gives you the passion to exert energy, momentum and intention into creating a new life from a new view point? You'll need to dig into your personal story to discover why you have the limitations you are currently living with.

There are two ways to approach this step:

- Write down your timeline of difficult events. Include how you noticed losing the possibility for greatness and wonder because of the event. (This method is tried and true. It's a bummer though because you are spending time with what's wrong. This process is not fun or glamorous, but it definitely gets the job done.)
- Write a full vision of how you would be if you were living your life at 100%, and identify what is different in your vision about who you are and how you are living now. (This second method is my preference. You'll find it a real eye-opener. You get to

operate from a place that assumes your awesome future has already been accomplished. You get to be the forensic detective identifying the dream killers.)

We'll go much deeper into perception as we work together. What is most important is to focus on your 100% outcome. You'll notice as you clear up a few key points that many others will automatically clear up, as well, because they were related to the first issue.

Here's the reason knowing your "why" is so important:

Once you've achieved a level of good health, wealth, and love, you may have less motivation to step it up to 100%. However, living with a perception that is not entirely yours means you are living an inauthentic life. It weakens your voice in the world. It weakens your power and your impact with others. As the new era supports naturalness and truth, moving into 100% living authenticity means you are seen as a leader in the global picture. Think about it: how many people do you know who live at 100% in any aspect of life? Imagine setting yourself into that special category of people who are living life, not only fully, but who are totally in charge of all aspects of their lives. In essence, you become the director of your own journey.

Maybe you already have a notion of the kind of impact that living at 100% functionality will mean for you. Honestly, very few people have ever really considered this was possible, so they have never dared to dream what a life full on, on your own terms, would mean.

You may have been on a good health plan or protocol for years, incorporating a healthy diet, exercise, and meditation among other things that help you feel good, but have you really considered a life without limits? Maybe you are afraid to have it all or to take a chance on yourself. One of my clients said working with me was the first time she had given herself permission to put herself first. If you don't take this step for yourself, love yourself, and improve your perception, you will always create and contribute from the "ground" of entanglements and "shoulds."

I think about this verse from scripture attributed to Jesus Christ: *"Love your neighbor as yourself."*

In other words, you must love yourself in the biggest way in order to give to others in the biggest way. "As within, so it is without." You cannot give more than you have. You cannot teach more than you know. You cannot live greater than the limitations you leave in your space.

The point is your 100% life is already within you waiting for an opportunity to be lived out to its fullest. All you need to do is take the first step. All you have to do is uncover, define, and clear away whatever stands between you and your vision of a 100% life. Then create a perception of your very best life, because that is what's already there for you to experience, and live up to the perception positions you have envisioned for your best life, the life you so deserve.

Everything is possible. There are no limitations; just endless possibilities.

✓ STEP 2: ESSENCE

The second part of your Divine Human Blueprint for restoring your unstoppable 100% life is your Essence. Take a moment and feel into your spirit. Spirit is you—your essence—that which comes with you, whether you are in or out of the body.

You don't have to be religious to understand the workings of your spirit. If you are religious or spiritual, what I am going to tell you next may surprise you.

Your Human Essence is comprised of three important elements: Human Spirit, Soul, and Life Force.

In the good old days, the only place you were going to hear about Spirit was in a church or temple. You had to knuckle down with your catechism or study for your Bat Mitzvah to glean the tiniest details about Spirit. If you were lucky, a priest or rabbi would take you under his wing and help you comprehend "human spirit"—that is, if they had a good grasp of it themselves. But truthfully, religion was not meant to teach you about the details of your personal spirit and its workings. Religion was, at its best, meant to inspire and direct an individual to the practice of communing with God. It is a beautiful practice when devotion, love, and prayer are combined to stir the heart to remembering its connection to God.

When it came to understanding your path in life as a human spirit, and the make-up of your essence, you had to trust the judgment and guidance of others. These individuals, perhaps church elders, were very likely no more an expert than you are in the workings of human essence.

Having found few answers in traditional religion, you may have sought outside your traditional religious training to gain more knowledge about human spirit.

Or you may have never really wondered about it at all. Most of the information available on the subject of human essence is outdated, fragmented, or only partially right. I have never seen the complete picture presented in one place.

Even if you were to make a study of human essence, with all the differing viewpoints on the subject, it could easily take you a lifetime to understand the importance of human essence and the role it plays in your overall liveliness and vitality.

The "Big Gate Keepers," the religious organizations throughout the world, determined what you would know about human spirit and what would remain hidden from your awareness. They created a group mind hypnosis to influence you to think that it would really be dangerous to fully comprehend your essence, knowing that you would shy away from your natural curiosity to know yourself well.

Think about all the folks in the 60s, 70s and 80s who swarmed to India in search of enlightenment. All these folks were on a quest, in search of their true nature. Ironically, they all adopted another culture and tradition in order to incorporate something different into their lives than what they had known from childhood. Still, the path of enlightenment was literally a path of moving away from bodily awareness and the mastery of the human experience towards a life of the spirit and the realm that is of spirit, which is accessed through meditation and prayer.

Joshua, who came to me after adrenal failure, asked me why all those enlightened masters he went to couldn't help him with his body. Why could no one heal him? The answer is that in order to be in a state of **enlightenment**, by most folks' standards, one must **reject one's physical nature** and hang out only in the higher realms of consciousness. Therefore, it was not uncommon for an enlightened individual to be sick, homeless, and broke.

This is not my idea of enlightenment. Nor would I seek after a transformation that does not point the way to full mastery of the human experience. How can you call yourself awakened, when your body is left in darkness to struggle, your financial situation is dire, and you will have to rely on social security to see you through your senior years? In this kind of "enlightenment," you have never taken the time necessary to know and love who you are or clear away that which is not you.

There is no longer a need to remain unaware. We are in the age of knowledge and wise-elder wisdom. You can now have the information that was once hidden.

Simply put, **Human Essence** is composed of the following three elements:

1. **Human Spirit** needing care and repair from time to time. Essence is, as described earlier, that which is with you whether you are in or out of your body. It is your light, your information, your presence.

2. **Human Soul**. We have in our culture mistakenly used the word, "soul," to describe spirit. Your soul is different than spirit. Your soul is the protective chalice of spirit. It is like a thick skin surrounding and protecting your light. It wanes or reduces in strength and size when you are unwell or under attack.

3. **Life force**. Though you might have imagined life force as part of your energy body, it does indeed belong in Human Essence. When your life force is low, you will feel weak. Simply by pumping your life force up using a quantum energy technique, your strength, vitality and energy can come right back. Literally, this reversal can happen in a matter of minutes.

Step 2 in the formula is the easiest to comprehend and certainly the simplest. As the song goes:

This little light of mine I'm gonna let it shine,
This little light of mine I'm gonna let it shine,
Let it shine, let it shine, let it shine!

Hide it under a bushel, no!
I'm gonna let it shine,
Hide it under a bushel, no!
I'm gonna let it shine,
Let it shine, let it shine, let it shine!

We'll get to the secret of keeping your Human Essence shining brightly shortly.

Once your life force, spirit, and soul are up to 100% expression, you will naturally have more energy, focus, and magnetism for living into the life of your dreams. Your mission and your blessing can then be shared with the world as your transformation begins.

The best part of "You Being 100% Human Essence" is that you can become brighter, clearer, and more focused. You can feel more energy in your physical body, and you can be attractive to what you are called to do. Being one with your essence does not require a third world visit, a priest's approval or a rabbi's sanctification. It's already part of you. You are the one in charge. You are in control. This, my dear friend, is a beautiful thing.

To ensure your light shines brightly in the world, daily meditation and the practice of appreciation and laughter are recommended.

✓ STEP 3: MATTER

Regardless of your personal or professional well-being, your life is worse when you are living a half-life and better when you are functioning fully at 100%. What you bring to the table regarding your work, love, vitality and your connections to others, is greatly enhanced by your vibrancy and 100% healthy body.

In this section we are focused on your body. You need to take a few steps up in the area of human matter and bring your best body—with its natural force, focus, clarity and momentum—with you to the game.

Matter is the human body, cells, glands, and organs, and the fluid, bones, and ligaments that form the body you live in.

Maybe you're saying, "But I am not very healthy. That's the way I've always been," or "I have diabetes or fibromyalgia and this part of the path is never going to get better for me," or "I'm cursed in love or business and nothing else has worked, so why would this?" etcetera.

Let me say this again. It doesn't matter what shape you are in, physically or otherwise. There are a set of principles, keys and practices that surround living in a human body. You were created with an accessible design and were meant to be able to "self-diagnose" and "self-restore."

You've just got to get the knowledge about your health and 100% life out of your head and into your being. My client, Alisa, who was an Immersion student, expressed her concern about having learned many modalities for healing, business, and relationships that sat dormant and virtually unused as she struggled both to support herself and get beyond a debilitating depression.

Learning to access your own Divine Human Blueprint, and becoming 100% healthy, requires no more learning. There is no next modality to learn, as the original Divine Human Blueprint is the whole kit and caboodle.

The choice is yours as to how you are going to work to improve your circumstances. You can turn your health and your challenges around to live a 100% life in sync with your Divine Human Blueprint. Or you can find more healers and healthcare folks to help you manage your symptoms or take yet another training to learn breakthrough strategies you already learned years ago and never could implement.

I use the term "could" here, because I want you to know that a lot of the blocks in your 100% life are not self-imposed. You have, literally, millions of programs running at any given moment in perception. In addition to perception, your DNA, which is a key part of matter, gangs up and gives you even more programs from family members. Imagine getting all the "loser" or "slave" programs from your ancestors. Ugh!

I'm going to say a strange thing here, so hang with me; I promise you will understand it in a few minutes.

You have to own your body 100%.

You have to then own and live in your body—cells, glands, and organs—100%. And finally, to really get to the place where you can be fully charged and powerful, you have to *be* the 100% healthy body. That includes your brain, nervous system, and all other systems, glands, organs, and every part of you that forms what we call, "matter." This is your ticket to freedom and a life fully empowered. Being in your 100% healthy body is necessary in order to realize your 100% potential

Using the Divine Human Blueprint, your body will be a primary source of joy and empowerment for you. You'll have the opportunity to up-level your health to the highest human potential. Feeling great all the time, and being able to access the 100% Healthy Divine Human Blueprint when something seems to be off, will give you an unstoppable and unending advantage in work, home, family, and love. Most importantly, your 100% healthy body will be the access point for going deeper into the fulfillment of your dreams. Wealth, fame, contribution, finding your soul mate, investing, running a marathon, becoming a marketing master, or becoming a bestselling author, whatever your big dreams are, they can only happen when your 100% healthy body can support your future vision.

Did you know momentum comes from the body? The forward movement of your momentum is accelerated by attuning your healthy muscles with a clear, focused mind. Suddenly, you are the mover and shaker. You're in the limelight and able to give life your fullest effort. You can generate momentum in all areas of your life and get up to par with the body in its prime.

Depending on your desires, you might choose to participate in an Ironman or Cross-Fit training competition. Or you might get up to mastery level with directed conscious reading. With your brain at 100%, you may be accelerating its speed by doing some brain plasticity exercises. (Brain plasticity was introduced by researchers in Japan years ago and increases both your ability to read quickly and the connections and communications of the neurotransmitters between the five brains—the instinctual, emotional, creative, logical, and genius brains, all housed in what we normally call our brain.)

You may find yourself in a "yes" mode that leads you to dive deeper into learning more about how love and relationships work. And now you have the momentum to fuel the journey in effortless ease.

If you are in charge of and "own" your physical matter (physical matter comprises all parts of your body), or if you are an entrepreneur or business person (or want to be), you have something very powerful to bring to the table. You can actually offer your gifts in tangible and manifested ways, because you are physically and fully present; you are really there.

Ideally, you would want your body at 100% optimal performance. I want to stress the idea of "100%," rather than the notion of perfection. Perfection tends to be a rabbit hole of deception and more a trick of the mind than a useful pursuit. Even when you are in the process of moving in the direction of your 100% life, you will be moving mountains and generating miracles in your world.

Turning your good health into great health is your best investment opportunity since you laced up your shoes, tied the bow, and went off to kindergarten to start your education. You wouldn't have the know-how to run a business or climb the "ladder of success" without a great education (some of which you continue to pick up along the way). In the same manner of "smarts" means "making money," "100% Healthy," or being your absolute best, gives you the foundation for fulfilling your mission and your vision at its highest level!

To get started, you will need to identify how you would like your health to improve. What are the areas that are already working well in your body? You may actually take these areas for granted; it's time to make a list of your assets. Survey your body. What are the areas your body is directing you to improve? Where do you want to have more vitality, high function, best chemistry, and strength in your physique?

Soon, I'll guide you through the process that will unlock your purely authentic, 100% healthy state of being. Together we can easily turn your body into your beautiful, biological, dream machine.

We start with what already works, while keeping a healthy perspective about the big picture. How are you supporting your body in attaining 100% health? You'll want to include exercise, drink large amounts of clean water, and maintain a good mindset through meditation and proper nutrition. It's also important to incorporate time to relax, as well as to work. Design an easy way to maintain your improving health and work it into your everyday plan. Once you've set the new standard for your foundational layer of support at 100%, you'll be ready to up-level specific aspects to your "matter." Improving DNA, the nervous system, adrenals and brain function may well be your next steps to attaining the state of 100% You.

There's a formula and a process for all of this.

The more proactive you can become in doing your activation meditations each day and following your Divine Human Blueprint formula, the faster you will get to the sought after space of empowerment, focused clarity, and juice! Remember, your magnificent health and the full experience of 100% health means magnificent manifestation and the ability to fulfill your dreams. There is no limit as to how deep you can go with the Blueprint to bring back lost luster and energy, and consequently, how far you can go in the world to fulfill your mission and generate your authentic wealth.

The more you practice being at the levels of 100% in all aspects of your Blueprint, the more being at 100% is reinforced everywhere in your life. For example, let's say you are aiming for 100% healthy rest and sleep. Then you notice that a natural side effect of having 100% healthy rest and sleep is that you feel brighter during your waking hours.

Once you bring your inner being—including your cells, your body and blood—into its fullest and best self, your outer world opens up. You can, with clarity, claim your outer world manifestations as perhaps a marketing genius, or a master healer, or whatever it is that you desire to create in your outer life.

But here's a quick piece of advice—pace yourself.

"If you want your dreams to be
Take your time go slowly.
Do a few things, but do them well
Heartfelt work grows purely.

If you want to live life free,
Take your time go slowly.
Slow beginnings, truer ends,
Heartfelt work grows purely."

(Thoughts attributed to St. Francis from the movie; *Brother Sun, Sister Moon*)

Don't let impatience or a "hurry up" mentality get the better of you. This can take you out of the game fast. There is enough time, energy, and love to get you back to you. By pacing yourself, you are telling yourself there is no emergency, that you are not on high alert, and that you will not be moving onto the next new thing if this doesn't work. Instead, you are living naturally with the knowledge that you are changing and growing healthier and younger with each passing day. You trust in the Universe. You trust in your body to restore itself.

This does not mean you should slack off from the 100% formula or stop working with your Divine Human Blueprint. I am talking more about maintaining an attitudinal adjustment. Get out of the "do or die" mentality and into the 100% healthy joyful lifestyle.

Once you have established great health, a positive mindset, and increased your energy, you will naturally go deeper into the fulfillment of your life's purpose and mission in the most meaningful and creative ways. You will be operating from a vantage point of being fully funded, and your own energetic field will support you like never before.

When you provide your body and mind with the right information and wellness patterns, you can take the next steps in your career and personal life. Repeat the processes of renewal using the Divine Human Blueprint formula as many times as you need in your quest to achieve your noble life, your life without limits.

Remember, your vitality and clarity are paramount. If you lose your vitality and clarity, or never restore them, you lose everything.

A 100% healthy you is built out of your original Divine Human Blueprint. This is the Blueprint that holds only your 100% healthy life-print as the guide. Capturing this original essence of a perfected you is simple and easy. Imagine a builder working off of a blueprint, but who never builds the home or castle the blueprint was designed for. Well, by ignoring the Divine Human Blueprint, which provides your instruction manual for operating the body, you are doomed to failure.

Using your blueprint literally guarantees success.

If you visit ***http://100YouBook.com*** *and watch video #3 in the free video training, you'll see an example of this formula at work. This video shows real people, who have gotten real results by using the 100% Healthy Divine Human Blueprint formula for restoring health, vitality, clarity, and focus.*

Feed your body with plenty of clean pure water, life giving foods, and happy moments that support your energy, vitality, and strength.

✓ STEP 4: ENERGY

Once you have the right mindset and emotions in place, your perception has shifted, you've gathered a possibly fragmented Spirit, Soul and reduced Life Force and brought it back up to 100%, and you've accessed the Divine Human Blueprint formula to restore all aspects of the physical body (matter) to its very, very best self, what's the next step?

The final step is all about getting your energy up to your peak performance.

You need energy. You always need to have energy fueling your body. And it's easy when you know the simple steps to make it happen.

You wouldn't believe how many times I have spoken to doctors and holistic practitioners, energy workers, and people who meditate regularly, all of whom have virtually no way to really return their energy and their energy bodies to 100%. They may have some technique they call a chakra healing or aura cleansing, but those barely touch the root of the energy problem. Although I applaud their efforts to connect with their energy systems, time and time again, their efforts produce no real, lasting results.

Back in the 1960s when flower-power was in and it was cool to have a guru to follow, hundreds of thousands of Americans made pilgrimage to the "Holy East" and hung out chanting and meditating at a guru's feet. Eventually they came back to their lives in the U.S. and filtered back into mainstream society, perhaps hanging on to a daily practice of meditation, or perhaps letting that fall away as they moved back into corporate and leadership roles and left their hippie days well in the past. They got a shot at mastering the energy body, since many of the teachers knew quite a bit about the chakras (energy centers), nadis (mini chakras), auras (energy field surrounding the body), and meridians (lines of energy running throughout and connecting the body).

Although they may have gained some knowledge, less than 5% of these practicing meditators actually mastered the wisdom of the energy body. Most never built the energy knowledge into the bridge linking the perfection of the 100% model of the Divine Human Blueprint to the physical body. They just didn't have the complete platform of knowledge.

Don't be that person. That's why "energy" is step 4 and not step

Let me explain a little better why energy comes now: If you have done activations for all of the previous three steps, energy will, and must, be the next activation

Earlier we spoke of perception. "In the beginning was the Word." Remember, much like our essence, perception defines how we will experience life. Although it does not have form, it is our intelligence, our "logos." From perception, human essence with spirit, soul and life force come into existence, and naturally must be restored to 100% light for your life to thrive.

Our spirit informs our DNA, even as we are cells dividing in our mother's womb, as to how to set up the game of life. Our life force activates, as we separate from our mother's life force at the time of our birth. Once perception and essence are made right, matter—the human body in all its complexity—must be addressed. Finally, our energy body, and the fuel we need to keep our physical body alive, is addressed. Energy is originally designed by spirit programming, sent into the DNA and grown after the body emerges from the passage of birth. The energy body develops largely in the first seven years of life.

Energy, the most advertised and sought after commodity on the planet, is natural and free—and for 97% of the population is elusive and confusing. Don't fall into the group of folks who keep their head in the sand and think that buying a six-pack of energy drinks is their way to sustaining energy. You are fully capable of accessing your 100% healthy energy system and getting yourself up and running for the best life ever.

When you have "PEME," you are just one letter away from the whole story, and with just this much information you can now, even without the last step, move into the most abundant, truly richest time of your life. Longevity is no longer something to study; it is something to live. Do you want to live youthful and beautiful for years and years, and decades to come?

The Divine Human Blueprint is a self-sufficient system that puts you in the driver's seat. You direct where your attention goes and how your energy flows. You live life on your terms—fulfilling your mission and manifesting your dream life. By following this system you move into the extraordinary 3% who "do" and "know."

Restore your energy. Your energy is your 100% lifestyle currency. With energy you can wheel and deal, speak to the masses, appear on TV, and run a marathon. You can fulfill the dream of deep love, and have the energy and love wisdom to sustain it for your entire life. Having energy changes everything. Pristine, bright, sparkly, loving energy is magnetic in the world. Want to get your message out? Sparkle up your energy. Want to feel authentic and credible, as you show people your system for doing something great? Then, my friend, let your energy sing with bliss.

To me, the magic starts when you reach the fourth step because energy fuels and enhances everything else in life. And the best part is that this is the easiest step to implement and access.

I know you are excited to get started. Later in our free video series, I'll explain how the different aspects of the Divine Human

Blueprint work and lead you in a guided activation to automate this entire process.

Now I've saved the powerful game changing part for last.

Having an attitude of gratitude is a game changer if you do it daily, because it keeps you in the flow of divine abundance. The more you appreciate and are grateful, the more the universe will match that energy and send you more to be grateful for. Set yourself at gratitude early in the day by listing 50 items you are grateful for. Be sure to include all the things that are working in your business, all the relationships you are in that are thriving, and include your amazing body (even if it is not yet where you want it to be).

✓ STEP 5: REALMS

It's time to add 100% energy, clarity, and wealth to your life and lifestyle right now.

My system is the only system that shows you the original, and ultimately the only, real way, back to living at 100%. You get there by accessing your own authentic Divine Human Blueprint and restoring your brilliance, light, health, and energy. Your Divine Human Blueprint shows you what to look for, how to leverage the good already in your life, how to make real headway in attaining the best of all worlds for yourself and your career and encourages you to share your newfound wisdom with the ones you love. The cool thing is the Divine Human Blueprint is already inside of you. You just need to understand it and bring it up to the surface once and for all. You, as your sparkly shining self—you, the authentic you—has not yet been introduced to the world.

(Some "100% You Formula" enthusiasts have decided to pursue a deeper path of activation in their 100% Healthy program. The Elite One Day and the Immersion programs are the best way in. The opportunity to be 100% is supported every step of the way. With more than twenty years' experience and thousands of happily restored individuals, the path is well-paved and ready to provide just what you need to effortlessly make your leaps up.)

The fifth aspect of the 100% Healthy Divine Human Blueprint is divided into four unique areas, each related to the other. You will see why we have them lumped together as I explain more to you.

The fifth aspect of the 100% Healthy Divine Human Blueprint is divided into four unique areas, each related to the other. You will see why we have them lumped together as I explain more to you.

The realms affecting humanity are unseen and powerfully influential. The four realms are (1) origin, (2) quantum, (3) amplification, and (4) embodiment.

Origin is where we came from and starts from the beginning of humanity. This realm dates back to original perception even before human spirit. This realm encompasses both historical and pure truth. It cannot be altered, as it just plainly "is." It is our guidepost and a true Omega. It is our record, our history of fulfillment.

Embodiment is what allows us as human spirits to take form in a human body. The normal way to experience the realm of embodiment is to be born to parents as an infant. Some yogis are able to move in and out of the realm of embodiment, taking their corporeal bodies with them into different fields of existence. They are also able to return, appearing the same as when they left us.

Quantum is the realm of connection, and oneness, with no consideration of time or space. Human mastery provides a powerful quantum field surrounding the master. It alters, bends, shifts, eliminates, and moves through time, space, health, wealth, love, and all things we can imagine. It includes all things beyond imagination.

Amplification is, in effect, like ripples emanating from a pebble thrown into a pond, yet far more powerful. In this expanding realm, not unlike our expanding universe, more is possible. This realm is related also to Genesis. It is spontaneous. It is a realm that is ultimately the precursor to energy.

Truthfully, you don't really need to know much about the realms to activate the Divine Human Blueprint and get yourself going in the direction of your "100% healthy, happy, wealthy, and in-love-with-your-life" life. The realms support the Blueprint as you may have already noticed. Most importantly, to understand the realms, take note if there is anything getting in the way of you having a full, rich relationship with each of the realms, in the area of perception. In other words, are you limited to being supported by just one of them or are you supported by all of them, based on programs in perception or elsewhere in the Divine Human Blueprint? If so, these are areas you will correct.

To me, the combined information of the realms is really the magic chalice that supports your healthy body and life.

Note: the more you activate the Blueprint, in other words, focus your intentions on the full experience of the 100% Healthy formula, the more rapidly things in your life will improve. Talk about walking around and sparkling! You will become a bright beacon of light, guiding all your dreams to you effortlessly.

The Divine Human Blueprint will literally kick-start your vitality, your career, and your love life, all at once. It will save you months or even years of struggle. Instead of going endlessly from one health practitioner, business coach, or therapist until you are overwhelmed with hopelessness and exhaustion., you will live and breathe in the light of blessedness and grace. How much is that worth to you?

Grapefruit essential oil is a wonderful energy tool. Use it in a diffuser in your work area to create natural clarity and renewed energy.

YOUR 100% LIFE AND LEGACY

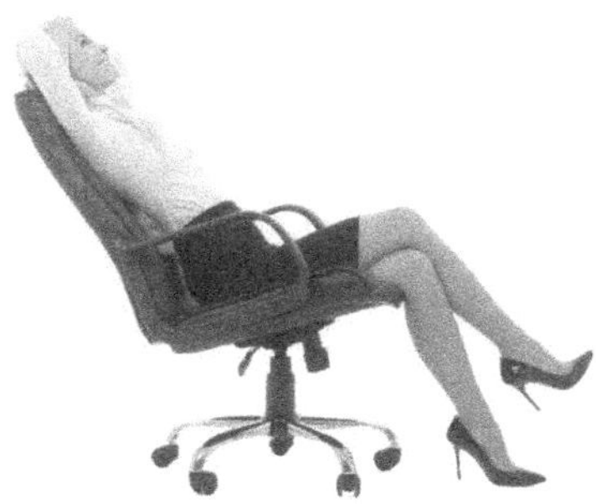

What You Will Want to Be Known For?

So, what is your foundational 100% health, wealth and love ideal? Match your ideals with your message and what you came into this world to accomplish. Why is it important for you to accomplish this? Why is it important for you to be living full out at 100%, feeling great, clear-minded and full of energy? What parts of your life don't support you in getting your work out into the world in the most powerful way? You need to determine your "why" and your "what." Understanding why you do what you do is a key part of this process.

What are you known for? How do people "read" you? Do they see you as vibrant? Full of crutches? Powerful? Weak? What do you want to be known for? How do you want people to "read" you? If you were to leave this world tomorrow, what would you want to be remembered for? What would you like to create as your legacy?

Now take a moment to think about your life and the stories from your own history that support your image of yourself as an innovator, and as one who thrives and overcomes impossible obstacles. List those stories with a few key words. (Reach in and find evidence. You have it in your nature to be a miracle maker.)

Here's an example to help you get started: I was told I would never walk without a cane, and later I was able to run 30 miles a week and dance on stage with a Rock & Roll band.

Now it's your turn! Grab your journal and put pen to paper. List a minimum of ten proof positives showing you are a miracle maker. Answer questions such as the following:

- What are your best attributes today?
- What were the highs, lows and the challenges you had to overcome along the way?
- How did you get through your health and business challenges to get to where you are today?
- What wisdom would you share with someone just starting out on his or her journey about what you have learned so far about life? Why?

The ultimate purpose of crafting your history is to enforce in your mind that you are a winner and to remind yourself that you can overcome challenges even when others say something is impossible.

You Are Not Living in a Black and White World.

You may believe the same ideas about health, wealth, and love that thousands of others believe, going along, while not consciously knowing that there is another more powerful way to be. But I promise you, every single person who I have ever spoken to about my own story of coming back from death, saying "no" to the Angel of Death, and choosing to live, even though medicine had no explanation for it . . . or growing back parts of myself that were surgically removed, and again having Western medicine tell me, after the fact, that I could not do that. Everyone who has heard my story has a knowing that there is more to life then the common group mind lives by.

So often I hear: *"I always knew that was possible; I just didn't know how."* You might be feeling that way right now.

Connecting with your emotions and your feeling body can help you get in touch with the truth of knowing that you can create what you want beyond what group mind says can be the accomplished or not. Trust in what you feel. Some people experience tingles or goose bumps, while others feel happy or excited. Still, others have a sense of experiencing a profound truth. When you get in touch with this profound truth—that life is more than what is seen or known, and more than what doctors and experts tell you—you can instantly move into the place of possibility. You can experience more of who you are and the perfection of your Divine Human Blueprint.

Parts of your story may be particularly difficult or challenging. You may not yet know why you chose to go through that experience (in other words, you have not resolved a painful experience by bringing it to a place of peace). Still, your uniqueness and the difficult episode that has yet to be resolved do not exclude you from the blessing and access to your 100% Divine Human Blueprint and the path to freedom.

The main reason we seek to resolve painful memories is so that you can restore a sense of trust—for your life, for the one you call God, and most of all, for you yourself, the designer and creator of your experiences. It's not about what "they" did to you right now; it's about how willing you are to free yourself from a painful interpretation of your history.

You must ultimately trust yourself to design a better life as you embark on the journey of accessing the Blueprint. The path to awakening your freedom and perfection has always been inside you. In your separation from truth, you have not been looking inside for the answers, but now you can.

What's Your Ideal?

- Self-expression?
- Health?
- Financial situation? Relationship?\
- Your message and legacy to the world?

And why do you want these things?

Clear your office and desk of the clutter. You may be able to function with stacks and piles of stuff around you, but know that this is wearing on your nervous system. You may not realize all this stuff undone keeps you in a state of high alert, pushing you to exhaustion and fatigue quickly. Let me explain a little more. Work that is undone sends a signal that you are incomplete. Too many incompletes can pile up in the unconscious and stress begins to build and impact the nervous system. If the only places you relax are out of the house or in front of the TV, you're impacted with too much energetic garbage.

KEYS TO THE KINGDOM

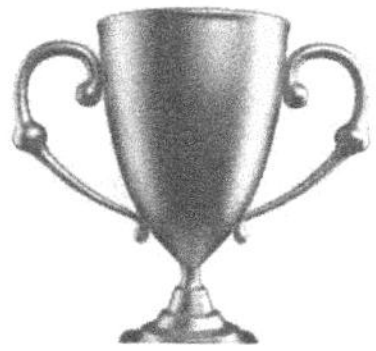

How to Automatically Access Your 100% Life

This would be a life with more vitality, energy and focus, to get you on your path to more love, money, better health, and a dream career where you have all your resources inside you already going at it and fully fueled to fulfill your legacy. Now, it's time to give you the keys to the kingdom.

I'm going to help you transform yourself into a "100% healthy—and-in-love-with-your-life—superstar" with a simple three-minute exercise. If you're already in good health, have money flowing to you, and are with the love of your life, I'm going to show you how to take your life from good to great and way beyond.

If, on the other hand, you have been sick and tired, struggling to get things to work in your business, or are holding onto old relationship baggage that is keeping you at a distance from the love and life you dream of, then prepare to be transformed.

Have you ever been afraid to fully want, dream of, or desire a 100% life, because you never thought it was possible, have no evidence to think it can be accomplished, or are afraid one more disappointment will be the straw that breaks the camel's back? Most people hold similar attitudes.

However, to dream the "impossible dream," so to speak, is the most effective and powerful way to create the connection back to your source information. By visioning what "could be," and making your vision larger than what the evidence of your life's experience or group agreement holds as "real," your connection with your authentic self is supported and enhanced. This is the self that is the one who knows the promise of a great life and that a Garden of Eden life is always possible

Your authentic self is this same self that magnetizes to you, love, wealth, health, and all the clients you can imagine. When you hold a big vision for yourself, it resonates with the ones around you, and their dreams become more possible, too.

Connecting with Your Source Code.

For generations we have been asleep to the fact that there is one definitive code that all humans are designed from. We skirt around it; perhaps the concept is too big or too scary to really embrace. If there is an original Blueprint or Source Code, then who designed it?

For now, let's put that question to rest. I promise to share details about the design in a future book about the access and deeper understanding of the complexities and intricacies of the design. For now, let us agree to know that the design is elegant, complex, and is meant to give us a grace-filled, incredible life.

This concept of an elegant design is a spiritually-based concept. In truth, I know this is factual because I have helped thousands of individuals access the design and reverse their challenges, as well as restore their health, wealth, love, and sense of peace in situations that appeared impossible. The transformation I speak of comes from your core. It is authentic and original and unique to you, as it is to each and every human.

The main obstacle has been one of unconsciousness and inattention to the Divine Human Blueprint. Perhaps we have all been just a little seduced into believing the powers that own the current database of knowledge (such as the scientific and medical communities). But if you leave logic to the side for a moment and check in with your heart and your intuition, you will find they will never steer you wrong.

Making the switch from mental information to authentic intuition is the secret to taking the first step back to your 100% healthy life. I am talking about a life without limitations. The more you access the Blueprint—especially in the area of perception—and clear what has stopped you, the faster you will get to your 100% life and lifestyle. The secret is to connect to yourself from a place that is authentic and innocent, because that's where new life begins.

For some of you, your BS meter may be going off. I promise that you will be agreeing with me soon. This works.

Imagine a light showing the way back to your authentic regenerative nature. What once was lost is now remembered. After eons of forgetfulness and disconnection from the source, where you were possibly lost in a world of pain, suffering, poverty, violence, or illness (which may have been followed by an assortment of pills, potions, and surgeries), finally, your Divine Human Blueprint, your origin, can safely be remembered.

I invite you to look at the strength of being able to refer to, and make renovations internally from, a builder's blueprint. Sagrada Familia in Barcelona is considered to be one of the most beautiful buildings in the world. This building is an exquisite, architecturally designed structure that could neither have been built or receive upgrades—renovations—without careful attention to detail paid to the structure laid out in its blueprint. To bust out a wall and not think it wouldn't affect the entire structure would be ludicrous.

Similarly, your life did come with an instruction manual. It's hardwired into your very being. PEMER, the system for understanding and accessing your Blueprint, is now available.

Think of it. We are in an era where you can consciously choose how to care for yourself. Leaders in the New Thought movement, like Louise Hay and Wayne Dyer, have all pointed in the direction of the Blueprint by making it popular to know and experience your life rather than be dictated to how to live. Christian Science says, "The body can and does know how to heal itself." T. Harv Eker tells us that we can "master the inner game of wealth." Anthony Robbins leads us into self-actualization and encourages us to maintain great habits in body, mind and spirit. Joel Osteen and Michael Bernard Beckwith point us in the direction of fulfilling our spirit's potential. Dr. Oz and Dr. Andrew Weil point us to a new approach to self-care, showing us how to cultivate healthy, happy bodies.

Let's face it. We live in an environment of readiness for the full knowledge of the Divine Human Blueprint to be remembered and accessed. We are ripe for the next steps. We are ready for the deepest awareness to be simply and naturally back in our conscious awareness for all to embrace and receive the benefits from this newly remembered knowledge.

Let me show you how to connect with your authentic design, how to have your Realms support your progress, and how to magnificently attract your perfect health, vitality, focus, wealth, love, and career into your life. This attraction skill will also make it profoundly easy to create new, better, brighter experiences in areas you've previously found yourself stuck in. As a bonus, this exercise will make you more comfortable in your own skin as well. Sound impossible? Well, let's see.

Stop using the computer prior to sunset. If you have trouble sleeping, this is a must. Staring into the bight screen can inhibit your pineal gland (the gland in your brain that is responsible for releasing the sleep hormone into the brain and body). In time, you may be able to return after leaving the computer during sunset to complete a project, but it's best to have no bright screens for 2 hours prior to laying down for sleep.

YOUR BEST LIFE

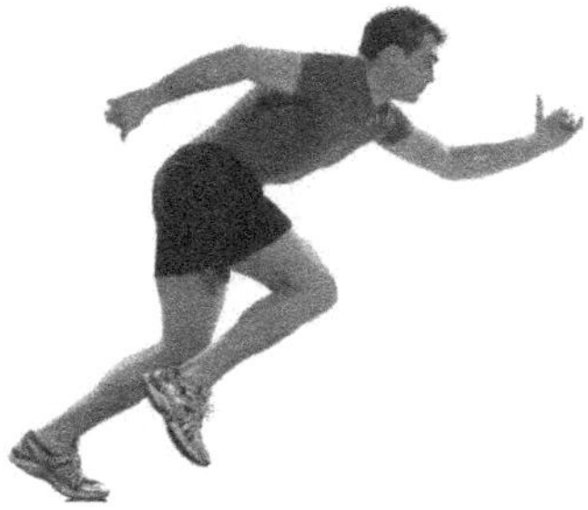

This exercise is called, "Put yourself first and foremost." In just a minute, I'll have you describe how it would feel to be your first priority.

At *http://100YouBook.com*, there's a free step-by-step video that guides you through this process, in case you're an "immersive learner" like me. Just "opt-in" and you'll get the printable, downloadable, "cheat sheet" companion to the video.

Remember a time when you were in the flow. You were unstoppable. It seemed everything you did turned to gold and you felt lucky, really blessed and happy. You may have to think back a ways, before "life" started to drain away your enthusiasm and energy. Was it a few days ago? A few years ago? Maybe a time in college or high school? Think of what you loved about life then. Who were you in this happy picture and in relationship to what you loved about your life?

It's possible you have only experienced these moments once or twice and consider it a fluke. So in this first step of the exercise, I want you to imagine being grateful, appreciative, and happy about your life. Imagine putting your needs before everything and everyone else; you come first. Imagine that you are the ultimate authority for everything that you choose and all that life brings you. By taking this first step, in which you are imaging a happy life where you are first and foremost in your life, you have begun to enforce your perception as a clear foundation for your 100% fully expressed life to manifest.

So, to manifest more of the 100% mindset in your PEMER, imagine your happy life. Write down a description of your ideal life in as much detail as possible. (Note: Do not worry if you are new to visualizing and dreaming and have no experience doing this,you can still effectively complete this exercise. I want you to just imagine your 100% happy, healthy, life.)

I'll give you an example: My client, Nancy, is an educator, turned entrepreneur. She shares custody of her two boys, and has an active travel schedule. She is thirty-nine years old, has concerns about her weight, about her mental clarity, and about getting her dream business off the ground. She is sensitive and loves people, but sometimes she becomes discouraged and loses her momentum when others rain on her parade.

Her dream life includes having momentum and vitality, having her metabolism at 100%, having a love life with a soul mate, having a booming career, connecting with her own tribe, and having a comfortable flow of money coming in. She also has been prone to fluctuating moods from hormones and a mild depression and wants to naturally stabilize her body chemistry up to peak performance.

Her greatest dream is to help others live a rich and fulfilling life while she travels and has fun, without having financial worries. That sounds good to me. How about you?

What I like most about Nancy is that she is eager, open and ready for more. She lives an enthusiastic life and is absolutely passionate about helping other people. By rallying that enthusiasm towards herself first, and then radiating that passion out to others, her imprint on others becomes so much more powerful.

The reason I enjoy working with Nancy is because she is clear that her health and vitality begin with her. She knows full well that she is the master and director of how she experiences her health, vitality, and her career success each and every day. When Nancy makes a commitment to step up and play in a bigger arena, she is right there, bringing her best self to the game.

Other people take themselves out of the game even before they begin. Fortunately, Nancy is a possibility seeker, who is willing to take action.

When I started working with Nancy, she was putting on a great show for everyone. She was using her positive attitude to lead with in her conversations, but there was no substance for people to grasp onto. She was the cheerleader rather than the master. Her words would land as inauthentic when her potential clients would listen to her conversations about how she could help them attain their dream life and financial freedom, because quite honestly, she hadn't found it for herself.

Nancy's quality of looking outside for the answer led her towards many different systems. She'd tried different coaching systems for her work and relationship life and couldn't implement them. When we worked together, she created total clarity about what she really wanted. (There is, by the way, what we want, which is based on what we think, and then there is what we, as essence, came into this world to experience; they are usually not the same.)

Nancy initially contacted me for a wealth clearing. We rapidly cleared her DNA and perception around wealth, and things in her life started to shake loose. She was booked for several talks immediately. Then a partner, who would have sabotaged her efforts, took herself out of the picture and some new clients appeared virtually without effort.

Within a couple of weeks, Nancy had new possibilities and a new plan. One flight-and-a taxi-ride-later, she was sitting in my living room for her next step. In Nancy's first "100% You VIP Day" we rebooted her brain, literally reestablishing 100% function in her master cells. (These are the oldest stem cells. Think of them like teachers; they teach the surrounding cells how to behave and how to function.) Then we cleared and restored her nervous system and adrenals to fully function.

What that meant for Nancy was that ease, focus, and clarity were restored, which enabled her to move into a big launch in her business. Her focus was so spot-on that her launch brought in thousands of new opt-ins. Her program for the launch was even better than all of her previous programs. And she gained the momentum to leave an unhappy relationship, lose weight, and move forward on all fronts!

The greatest wish that I have for Nancy is that she experience 100% satisfaction and 100% performance in all areas of her life. She loves the notion of automating her income and bringing in big money through summits and speaking, and I am watching her move at lightning speed toward her goals. With her clear focus and mastery in marketing, I could see her making money, feeling purposeful, living fully, and impacting people who resonate with her message.

The possibilities for her health, happy hormones and great metabolism were also fulfilled by accessing the same Divine Human Blueprint that brought her love and money. Nancy living her mission in joy and celebration is my best vision for her.

Done. When you follow this process, you'll access your 100% life and lifestyle just like Nancy.

Got it?

Exercise:

Step 1: Describe "Your 100% Life" —the best life you could ever imagine. (If you are new at this, then IMAGINE how the things in your life that do not work currently will be when they work at 100%):

- What benefits will you experience when your brain functions at its best, so that you feel clear focused, and energized, instead of in "deficit mode"?
- Think of someone you loved. Notice how you felt when you were in love, and how it feels when you imagine loving yourself and putting yourself first. Fill yourself up first so that you can love your partner at the deepest level.
- What might happen if you align with wealth, and have all negative perception related to having wealth cleared? Can you visualize your flow of money improving as you attain, grow and sustain your wealth?
- Imagine your results from accessing the "100% Healthy Divine Human Blueprint." Can you visualize yourself as healthy?
- Can you see your clients attaining their best results?
- Who is raving about your excellent performance, your athletic abilities, or your contribution to the team effort?
- What would it be like if you could put an end to a chronic condition, such as asthma, allergies, chronic fatigue, sleepless nights, PMS, fuzzy brain, rashes, hair loss, etc.?
- Who are you when all is working well in your life, and you are feeling enthusiastic, warm, happy, sharing, caring, and fun?

Okay, it's time to take out your journal and get writing! Go ahead. Don't skip this. It will be fun!

Step 2: Now do the following (this is really easy!): Close your eyes and imagine you are rooted to the earth. See a field of golden energy around you. (Congratulations, you are now accessing your quantum field). Take a deep breath in. Exhale. Smile deeply and feel the glow around you beginning to build. Imagine any dark colors that are in your field flowing down through your roots. Continue to breathe in and out, feeling your breath fill your heart and lungs. Breathe in even more deeply. Now you can breathe down into your belly and pelvic cradle. Keep breathing in through your nostrils and breathing out through your mouth. Smile.

Now think about the best feeling you have ever felt in your body.

As you imagine this peak body experience, notice that you begin to actually re-live the feelings you had back then. As you feel the waves of peace, bliss or excitement wash through you, use your inner gaze to begin to see your 100% life.

In this life, you are surrounded in love, your health is incredible, and you have the best clients ever. Feel fully fueled and grounded in the feelings of great gratitude and love.

Now we're going to imagine the story of your transformation to 100%. Simply and easily see the field of golden energy around you supporting your effortless process as you blissfully love and appreciate everything building in your beautiful world. Your magnetic field and your vision come together as the circumstances of your 100% life seem to build and expand. Access to your quantum field is open. Your bank accounts are overflowing, love embraces you, and everyone you know is commenting on how amazing you look; you are so energized and youthful. You smile to yourself, filled with passion, gratitude and enthusiasm.

Note: *I want you to feel. Be emotional. This is not a mental exercise. Feel into your nature and feel into your heart. This is your feeling exercise.

So take a moment now and record the images and awareness you experienced in this transformative state.

If you really felt into this exercise, I can guarantee that your journey to 100% has begun. If you imagined the momentum and energy fueling more clients, and bringing in more money and love for you, and you felt into it, leaving your thinking mind out of the vision and allowed your feeling perception to act as captain, you have reset your perception to a new, and much higher expression of yourself.

Accessing your quantum field is not done by the means of thinking; it is done by presence. Let me explain.

For the past five years, I have taught my Immersion students (we used to call the program by a different name) the technical aspects of the Divine Human Blueprint. They would get their hand moving to a simple pattern I taught them and start working on projects by thinking their way through the process.

Even though I would tell them their energy needed to match that of love and appreciation, they would routinely overlook that instruction, skip this step and jump to technique. These were intelligent folks, among them doctors of science, medicine and theology. Actually, they were BIG thinkers and they would literally beg me for more and more details to the Blueprint. Though many were successful in accessing the Divine Human Blueprint and making shifts for themselves and others, I personally felt they missed out on the real journey. Accessing the Divine Human Blueprint is a simple journey, a journey into self-love and self-awareness.

When you come to the Divine Human Blueprint from the space of love—no matter what you were thinking or feeling before—this self-love and self-awareness opens the door for you to access what you need for your corrections and activations.

These processes lead you back to 100% you.

This is the key: You must stay in the space of **LOVE** to open the door. You must be determined to be a 'love ambassador,' loving yourself first, than loving others from fullness. Joy and enlightenment are also access points for the Blueprint, but for now let's stick with LOVE.

How did your exercise go?

From this point forward you have opened the possibility for a life that can be lived at 100%. Through the process of imaging, you have set your perception to a higher standard and your life is beginning to transform.

Remember not to overstress and struggle. Just do your best and continue to make shifts up as you feel room for more. Living a wealthy life means living in balance and ease. At some point when striving and driving forward get to dominate your every action, it is time to step back and remember how we were meant to enjoy life. Too many tanks empty and you become run down and exhausted.

REVITALIZATION AND RESTORATION

Begin by REVITALIZING One Area and RESTORE Many Other Areas in the Process

It's only a little counter-intuitive, but if you get one area of your Blueprint up to 100%, other areas will naturally rise in the process.

If you attempt to do all areas at the same time, you actually won't get a great result anywhere. A big mistake is to try and fix a big bunch of problems and challenges all at once. When you do not get specific in your clearings, you miss important details. You will want to follow the directions laid out here as you begin to improve your programs in perception.

This is not wishful thinking or imaginary "woo-woo." I urge you not to approach this like the gambler who is placing all his bets on a big win. It's the wrong approach entirely. *Grounded belief* is fueled with authentic gut feelings of knowing and truth.

From this perception, your progress is catapulted. On the other hand, the gambler's attitude loses all power by leaving out the elements of personal responsibility and personal accountability.

I would rather you pace yourself slowly and steadily, and educate yourself, spending time learning about yourself and the improvements to your life that will most benefit you than for you to throw your hat in the ring and demand of yourself: "Okay, I've waited a lifetime for this; I want it all right now!"

It's not realistic. The Divine Human Blueprint is so much more powerful than magic. I promise you. And you can, and do, already access it.

I want to share a few more details with you about my story, and how I first started experiencing the magnificent transformations from the Blueprint.

I mentioned I had come to the end of my desire for life on earth due to the level of pain and suffering I was enduring each day. My doctors had given up on any possibility for a good life for me. The weeks before my garden experience were rough. I had cervical cancer, and while in surgery, they discovered how sick I was inside. They took my uterus, ovaries and cervix in that surgery, (and that is the last surgery I will ever need).

After that surgery, all of my doctors began to treat me as a hopeless case. Previous to surgery, my surgeon had told me I was imagining the pain in my belly. He said he would take pictures during surgery so I could see I was imagining the whole thing. When I awoke, the surgeon was in shock. He looked empty, (his usual cockiness had disappeared). I had a strong sense from his demeanor that unconsciously he was asking me to comfort him. There were no surgical pictures produced. When I asked him about them, his response was, "No, it was too messed up in there."

Twelve days later, I hemorrhaged and was readmitted, having lost a lot of blood. This is where a group mind virus can get started. (You may have had a group mind virus hold you in stasis despite your efforts to shift to a new position. It feels like an imaginary impassable wall and it defines a lower level of function, whether in business, love, or health.)

I have always been intuitive, clairvoyant actually, and the three treating physicians were all sending me death thoughts. What I mean was that they had seen something they did not understand. I looked like a normal woman on the outside (one in a lot of pain). But on the inside I looked like I had survived Hiroshima. The recurring thought I heard was *"if your womb is that bad, imagine what your heart, lungs, stomach, kidneys, liver, and spleen must look like."*

Perhaps they didn't know how to handle this knowledge, or perhaps this was a way for them to resolve my imminent demise in their minds. Whatever the case may be, I do not fault them for not knowing what to do or that their thoughts were actually harmful to me. When I said they did not believe in my possibility, I mean literally—all of them in their minds were showing me that I would soon be dead. So loud were their thoughts that my psychic friends warned me: their thoughts were dangerously affecting my field and I needed to move away from the treating doctors if I wanted to live.

Okay, so now I have shared with you what I was up against. Hopefully, you are not sick or struggling, but whatever your current state of health, love, or financial security, I am sure you can relate on some level to what I am talking about. Have you ever felt someone in your space so loudly telling you that you cannot succeed, that it overrides your best intentions?

I was at a weird impasse. I couldn't look to traditional medicine for help to get well because they didn't believe I could. Yet, I had no real options as to how I was to get better. I had already tried every alternative medicine in the book, and although I would often experience some improvement or at least some relief, I was not turning my dire health condition around in a big way. In fact, I was getting worse.

One thing I have always known is that I am a beloved child of God. I always knew my friends, Jesus and Mary and other avatars, loved me. I felt their presence, saw them, and had interacted with them since early childhood. I'm sure you've heard of very ill people having had visions and revelations. I personally believed that this message from Jesus was meant for us in this age to hear:

> *"This and even greater works than these you shall also do."*
> —Lord Jesus Christ

Are you familiar with this message?

I felt in my heart of hearts I was promised a good life, a life free of pain and suffering. I believed it, like an innocent child. The part that had been missing to make this real for me was that I didn't have my perception set for 100%. Quite the opposite: I was set to survive, to overcome, but not to reverse the damage. Something came to me that week, an idea, a gift for a new perception. It was the strong promise of a good life, one without suffering. I began without knowing consciously that I could reset my perception to a new level. I didn't know about setting anything to 100%, but I did know my suffering had to end.

Revelation in the garden

I brought my best self to God in the garden that first day, and all the days thereafter. I bathed, wore silk, carefully put my home in order, and sat with a puja tray in which candles and incense rested, lit for the day. I learned Bhakti yoga in India; this is the yoga of devotion. How perfect. I sang love songs to God till my heart was bursting with love. My quantum field was expanding and love permeated my inner garden like never before.

Love opened the door to the first of many access points and up-leveling shifts. For years, I called these up-leveling shifts of physical function "miracles." Isn't it funny; our culture puts miracles into the category of unexplained magic? Yet five years after my garden transformations, the science and medical professionals sought me out, asking me to share with them the secrets from the Divine Human Blueprint.

Eventually, I was able to translate the experience and break down each process into easy-to-understand scientific terms that could be replicated by people who did not share my faith. I realized the Divine Human Blueprint was, indeed, meant for everyone.

The access gateway to both the Divine Human Blueprint and the quantum field is love; it is the key, the secret that was never meant to be secret.

After years of improving my own design, I finally made a decision. I said to myself: *"I am going to live 100% healthy, happy, in love, wealthy, and connected."* When I tested that statement using muscle testing as to whether or not I believed this affirmation to be true, I found resistance in perception from both others and myself. In other words, my perception provided some negative programs. Combined, these programs ran continually. They included the build-up of beliefs related to my imminent death, the need for struggle, poverty, servitude, and many other issues All of these thought forms, mostly from others, dominated my perception. The good news is I found a way to easily address these impediments and move forward. Because of this, I am now literally experiencing the healthiest, happiest, most successful time of my life.

Having attained this level of fullness using the Divine Human Blueprint, and having recently discovered the secrets to getting there easily by using perception to clear away obstacles prior to working specifically on an issue, it is now the perfect time to invite you to join me on the journey of self-actualization, manifestation and awakening to your best ever, 100% life! I believe in living my life purpose, and what gives me fulfillment is to help you. I came here to not suffer, but to remember. I came to share love with you. If this message resonates with your spirit, if it sounds exciting and right to be your 100% best YOU, and if you can feel it in your bones—then I welcome you with open arms to join me. Let's go for the gold and "'do" 100% together.

Limit your time on social media, perhaps to a half hour daily or even less. It is great to communicate, however social media can be a real time vortex. Understand that when you are on the Internet you have gone into a trance state. What this means is one of your brain waves has turned off and you are more easily influenced. You go into a state similar to the addiction of chemicals. You are not in present time on the Internet; you are in "Machine Jurisdiction." There are no good boosts that come into the higher levels of brain function from this place.

YOU CAN DO THIS

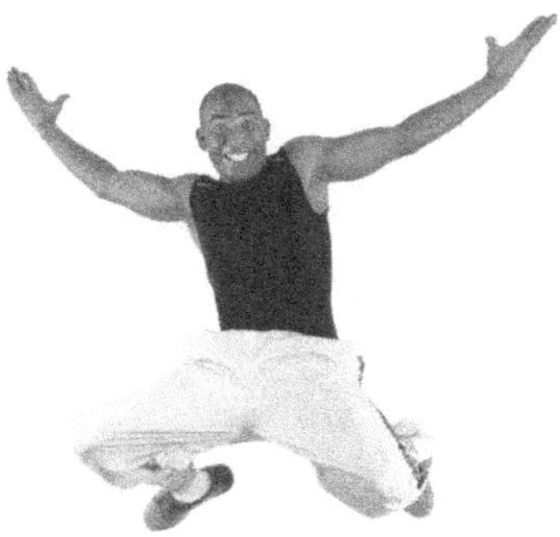

I invite you to go to your bathroom mirror and repeat after me: "I CAN DO THIS."
You can.

Want proof? Several years ago, after working on honing my skills with the Divine Human Blueprint, I began teaching students how to activate their own 100% healthy life and lifestyle. Please understand this information is for everyone with a human body. It works for people who have the most difficult challenges, as well as for people who need some simple tweaks in order to shift from good to great.

At an event last spring, I crossed paths with a dear friend in the MLM speaking industry, who shared with me that she thought the economy had ruined her business and that she hadn't been booked to speak for months. After tuning up the cells of her brain, we reset her perception, removing the group mind around 'her' bad economy. I kid you not; she immediately booked two paid speeches and her chemically-based depression cleared.

Tyler, a handsome, dark-haired, younger fella, who was Internet savvy, found me on YouTube. He had spent countless hours daily searching for a cure for his adrenal failure. Like a mouse in a trap, no matter what he did, he was confined to home and he'd struggled, living as an invalid, virtually bed-bound for 5 years.

Tyler had come across a video of Holly, who while being treated for a serious illness, began using the principles of the quantum energy focused into the Divine Human Blueprint and was experiencing incredible results. On her initial PET scan, she was told she had one nonfunctional adrenal. A short four months later, the PET scan report showed a fully functional, full-sized adrenal.

The possibility of adrenals really healing gave Tyler hope. Maybe he, too, could get better. And sure enough, within three short months from the first "Elite 100% You" one-day activation Tyler did with me, his adrenals became fully operational. He is now exercising and out of bed. It's a big transition for him, as he never really held down a job before, or experienced life as a healthy adult.

Now, Tyler is working with my wealth program (Accelerate Wealth) which will help him discover what he is here to do in the world, now, in present time.

I've mentioned two individuals who were suffering from the worst of health with very bad adrenals and physical stress. These same principles work really well for the **superstar**, the over-working entrepreneur, who is busy getting on as many stages as possible. Avoiding burn out and knowing a few simple steps to keeping both the adrenals and the nervous system clear are incredibly empowering. If I am describing you, please visit **http://JulieRenee.com/FTF** for a free 5-day course on improving adrenal health.

If you are experiencing either love or money challenges, you will be thrilled with the activations from the Divine Human Blueprint and how they can positively affect your outcomes.

Ever notice how there seems to be a lucky few—people who are incredibly fortunate and who have things always go well? Then there are the others who take the same action, yet get a completely different and less than desirable result. Ever wonder why?

Perception allows us to define or affirm positive words of what we wish to create, but our words are influenced by negative group mind. Negative group mind exists outside the constructs of the human brain, authored by you in the ethers.

For example, imagine all of your own originating thoughts in perception, then add to your thoughts things people have thought towards your group, or you, as a whole being. An example of this would be my three doctors, who held a strong group mind connection, where at one point, all thought I was going to die. Their thoughts turned into form and became an influencing factor in my perception.

Don Miguel Ruiz, author of *The Four Agreements*, talks about this kind of thought form as black magic.

Surprisingly, it is easily removed. The most important factor is to be aware that the negative thought forms from group mind exist at all. To free yourself from this problematic programing in perception, you must be aware there is a block in perception. To successfully remove this issue, you don't need to know the details. Just apply the principles of clearing, which by the way, involves a very simple technique using the same hand movement I teach to clear perception programs. Using this technique, you will successfully and rapidly remove this impediment.

I started out by using the principles of Quantum Activations with the Divine Human Blueprint to improve my own my health, wealth and money experiences before working with others. Essentially accessing the quantum field, I am able to direct this regenerative energy into the problem area, and by using the Healthy Divine Human Blueprint, I am able to bring into manifestation the 100% version of that which was previously defeated and sick. After I mastered how I was getting the changes to happen rapidly, I designed a course and taught a yearlong program, geared for those already in the healing and wellness professions. My students learned how to take this blessing out into their respective communities, and with their followers, share this incredible transformative system.

Melany is a perfect example of taking the activations to the next level. I met and worked with Melany at a live event. When I was with her the first time, one thing stood out like a flashing red light—her brain was not working well.

She had experienced brain trauma resulting from a concussion while doing gymnastics as a child. If you have had a concussion, the brain does not go back to full function, unless you activate the Blueprint. Melany, now age 40, well-spoken, successful and very personable, actually knew that there was something really wrong, and when I told her we could get her brain back to 100%, she was thrilled.

We did several 100% Healthy one-day sessions and brought her brain way up!

Now, to the outer world, she already looked and functioned as a healthy woman. She is a competitor who loves cross fitness training. For Melany, it made sense to tweak her insides to 100% to match who she presents herself to be so she would be in sync with her best performance level in both her inner and outer world.

What I loved about Melany was her commitment to follow through. If she had a headache, she would text me to learn the proper approach to clear it. If something was off, she would ask me to help her dig down to discover why, and then, she would work on her own corrections for the situation. She is not a health practitioner, or a scientist; she is an openhearted woman who lives in the possibility that she can experience 100% in all aspects of life. Bravo, Melany, bravo.

It takes a mindset shift, or really a shift in perception, from the fast food mentality, which directs you to find a quick first answer outside yourself, to *'it's important for me to go inside and discover what is off so I can correct it once and for all'*.

What I am seeing is a shift among my following from a formerly large group of people, who were very ill with chronic and terminal illness, to my present time clients—a new group of conscious, awake individuals who are already experiencing good health and success and who want to live the fullest, best life they possibly can. It is the ambitious entrepreneur, the one who refuses to play small, who is now plugging into the quantum shifts provided by the Divine Human Blueprint. The Blueprint gives them more than a slight edge—not just over their competition, but over their lower-functioning former selves.

It's time for you to let go of the "dreams deferred syndrome." Having this syndrome means you are too exhausted or unfocused to carry out your mission in the world. Let's agree to a new way and embrace a new rebooted life where you are able to fully express yourself with vitality and clarity.

When I first started talking about the Divine Human Blueprint in my practice, and showing by example how to experience improvements, the very sickest people came to me in hopes of a miracle.

What I began to see very clearly is that if we can get to you before the problems set deeply in, you can remain in charge of your health. You can move into your future without the overwhelming potential for a tragic illness—at least, you can get a deep hold on your own design and live your healthy, happy life.

For two years, I offered a very time intensive, yearlong program for creating miracles. This intensive was attended by the very ill. In the course, people were thrilled as their dreams for health resurfaced. They could see real physical evidence, evidence that wow-ed their doctors and showed everyone that their lives and health were becoming dramatically better.

Enlarged prostrates shrunk, broken bones mended on the spot, illnesses and pains cleared up, hair grew back, vitality returned.

Yet, these folks had such strong perceptions rooted in suffering, and their identities were attached to how bad some things were.

Regardless of the many improvements each of them was making, I found them, as a group, difficult to work with. Although there were a few positive, happy people in the group, their negative storytelling would diminish their cell regeneration and would defeat the positive momentum we were bringing in.

Then it occurred to me: work with healthy people. Get to folks before there was a lot to weigh them down. That is when the "100% VIP" one-days and the "100% YOU Immersion program" came into being.

The 100% Healthy Elite one-days are producing the results I always knew were possible. Together, we get your brain, nervous system and hormones right. When all systems are set to go, watch your world open up. Hand in hand, the physical upgrades lead the way to a financial or love upgrade. Getting to 100% in one area of your life stimulates growth in other areas. The system is meant to build off of itself, and as the body gets better perception, your essence and energy get better, too.

As the work with the Divine Human Blueprint builds and moves out into to the world, I can see discussions and important conversations taking place on national talk shows. Wouldn't Oprah Winfrey love this stuff? Perhaps the *Today Show*, Dr. Oz, and Dr. Phil could add to the conversation in intelligent and meaningful ways.

I've always thought Deepak Chopra tuned into the same golden light waves that I tune into, as his topics would echo my blog and radio shows, as if we were somehow tuned to the same cosmic satellite station.

What would be really cool is to have Suze Orman, the money guru, address how perception, when shifted, makes your money picture better. Or the relationship expert, Alison Armstrong, who could speak about the new freedom that can be found in a relationship after removing the stuck entanglements from your perception.

You're probably just starting to comprehend the far-reaching shifts to your very being that can develop by accessing your Divine Human Blueprint. You can improve the simplest things, like instantly clearing a headache or cramps, or work on something that feels more complex, like freeing up a problem in your aura of being a "servant," so you can be the powerful leader you imagine yourself to be.

All of these clearings are simple and easy. These issues, and many more, can be cleared with little more than the wave of your fingers. Abracadabra, presto change-o, and there you have it.

Although it looks like magic, it only looks that way because the entire population forgot this information. But amazingly, it is wired into your very nature.

I have to stress this is not a new age "deal-ly-bob" or an "airy fairy" notion. I've worked with the BIG technology guys, and as I mentioned earlier, I've worked with people at the Pentagon, the United Nations, and a whole lot of rich and famous people, and they have no qualms at all about availing themselves of the incredible benefits and results from accessing and activating the design.

Now, together, we're putting an end to the Divine Human Blueprint being the best kept secret on planet earth. I am here to love and support you, be a beacon of light, and to get the secret for living 100% into your hands. It's my reason for being.

I may not know you yet, still I feel confident that if you were given the choice to live at 50% and continue to degrade to much less, or choice two, to live at 100% and keep yourself feeling awesome for years to come, you would choose the path of grace and ease.

This is the power of clarity. Imagine getting so clear about the fact that you are meant to live in an amazing, healthy, happy, vibrant state and that anything less will just not work anymore. Instead of taking the slow path to your best life ever, taking years or even lifetimes, you can choose to live it now. No more waiting.

Just like me, you can shift up to 'UNRECOGNIZABLE HEIGHTS.'

Right now.

The process of creating is God's gift of healing through our essence: leaving the mind out of the equation, we can move out of that which has settled in the body.

A PROFOUND SECRET

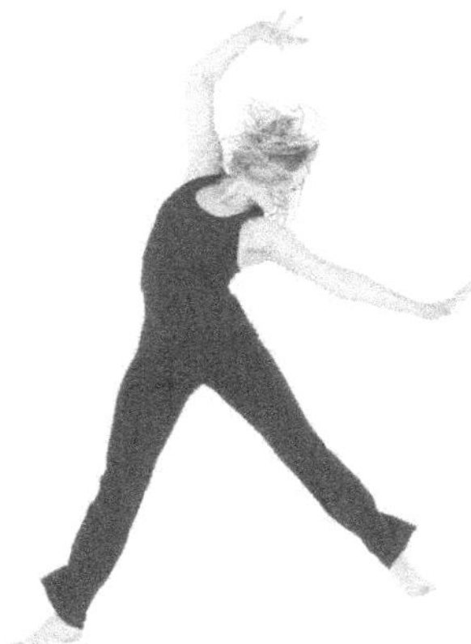

Instill the concept into your perception that you can, and are, meant to live at 100% feeling great in your body. Living full on and following your purpose is the ultimate secret to living at 100% and is truly your first step.

You may be used to looking at people, understanding what holds them back, but you may not be so good at looking at yourself and identifying your own blind spots. Honestly, most people find it much easier to see where someone else is stuck, than to see their own issues. So the trick to getting into the 100% experience is to begin by noticing every time things are not at 100%, and agree with yourself that it is possible to have this area of your life be at 100%, too. I know this may actually seem a bit redundant, and simple, but this is the most important thing you must open to.

When I was pregnant, sick, and dying at age twenty-four, I prayed that God would save my son. I prayed to survive the pregnancy so I could give him a life, even if I could not be there to raise him.

I carried him through till his due date, and he was born healthy, pink, and was eight pounds. At the same time he was entering the world healthy, pink and full of zest, I weighed in at 104 pounds. I was frail, green, and too weak to walk.

Had I known then what I know now, I see I could have been healthier than ever at the time of his birth. But the programs I had installed in my consciousness from what my doctors told me was that I would ultimately not survive. My perception programs were telling my physical body it would ultimately not survive this illness and that death was imminent. So the thought forms of death were dominating my psyche.

Six months later when I died for the first time, I looked down on my body, and watched my life flash before me. I said, "No, God, I don't want to leave. I have purpose; help me survive." I did survive... just survive. I hadn't really shifted perception enough to start really taking on life fully.

Will 17 surgeries, multiple cancers, a year in a wheelchair and 5 Near-Death experiences improve your perception? Yes, and no. Yes, in the sense that what I felt was that every day was precious. But no, because in my mind, I thought my life and illness would always be a struggle, and that I would always have to fight for my life.

What I now know is that my life and my health are always my choice. I get to choose. I set and clear away perception elements. It's my menu. I don't need to survive if I want to thrive. I don't need to live in the reality of "thrive," (which on my scales reads about 70%) when I can live in bliss, completely healthy, energized and alive, fully funded, and deeply in love.

Feel into your beliefs now. I want you to appreciate yourself for any of the tough things you lived through. It is an extraordinary person who gets their innocent outlook back after something difficult has happened.

I want you to take inventory as to where you are with perception. For example, if you went through a bad divorce, how do you now imagine love? Do you focus on what you definitely don't want, or on what would work for you? Or perhaps you have said, "I'll never do that again; it hurts too much," and have left the possibility for real deep love in the dust along with the rest of your dead dreams. What is your choice?

Here's the bottom line: You've got to awaken the dreams of your 100% life that have been lying in ashes. Raise them up, just like the phoenix, to live brightly anew.

Okay, I hear you: "But Julie Renee, if I could have done that, don't you think I would have already? I have two answers to that comment:

1. You may never have really looked at the possibility of revitalizing your dreams, so you may never have even tried, or

2. You likely have never activated your Divine Human Blueprint to 100% possible. So even if you had tried, without clearing perception, all the thought forms that exist in conflict with your 100% life fought you.

I know you can relate to this. Think about all the times you committed to a "new you." Using your best intentions, you knew you could change. Then you lost the possibility of change, and even to you, it looked like you were self-sabotaging.

I have news for you. Although you may not have kicked in with will to strengthen your resolve, you actually weren't sabotaging; you were attempting to bring in new and better pictures for your 100% life but hadn't yet cleared the old garbage away. How successful would you be in building a symphony hall on top of a city dump?

There were a whole lot of years I didn't want you to know about how sick I was, and how bad things were for me. I was afraid you might not respect me. Or worse, you might have questioned how in the world I could know anything about being 100% when I had spent years of my life (literally) in a hospital bed taking crazy amounts of medication? I know that I am not my past. I am not the old body or that with former health issues.

I choose to not hide from you and to let you really see me, raw and exposed, and fully in my dignity. By sharing what went off in my world, you and I now have a deeper connection.

If I had the courage to fight all those years for my life, I believe your getting the secret to living a life of much greater **possibility** (without all the drama and bad times) makes sense. I want you to benefit from my lifetime and the wisdom I've gleaned. I'd love for you to get to your possibility without devastation.

For years, I was worried I wouldn't be alive long enough to get my legacy out to humanity. Now, that worry has evaporated into nothingness. I have a long life ahead with endless possibilities.

My legacy is your legacy.

As I move away from the stress around getting the knowledge and awareness of the Divine Human Blueprint out into the world, I relax and can see my weaknesses and clear them.

Not knowing anything about how to market my information about the Divine Human Blueprint was a stop. But when I cleared spaciousness and created a long life in perception, I was able to make room to learn how to become a master marketer.

You may have studied with some of the greats in marketing. There are so many. However, you may not have been able to really integrate or implement what you learned because you had blocks in perception.

Until I shifted, I could hear everything that was being presented, but I would feel tangled up inside, frayed, and nervy. I would push myself to create a result, but with so many issues in perception, I could rarely really win. I am so grateful to the master marketers in my world in present time, who are helping me learn marketing relevant to today's audience. As I clear away the blocks, I can truly become a master at anything I set my mind to—and so can you.

I have also found in my work that women, especially ambitious leaders or those who are striving to be leaders, put on a great face to the world, but are hiding the truth about their internal workings to everyone. They are aware of problems, but manage the problems so no one really finds out the extent of the issues.

I get it; I soooo get it.

But I'll tell you what. You may be able to cover over your challenges to the world for a while, but at what cost to you? If you are not in great shape, how can you bring your best self forward? What is so important that you would ignore your health, sleep, fatigue, hormones, fuzzy thinking, and exhaustion? You can likely add more to this list. So my question is: Why do you do it?

Twenty years ago, I predicted we were entering an age where the true value of a person would be based on his or her contribution and impeccability. In this time, we would become transparent and we could feel into others. We could see if a person was being true to their word and if they lived what they spoke. The importance of money and possessions would be secondary to a truthful life.

I know we are in the beginning of this era as I see how transparency is becoming more and more important. People want to feel and relate to a real person, not a fake-pretend person. I want to know you, really, the real you. I want to be inspired, not just by what you say, but by how you make me feel when I am with you. This is where the power and the wealth are.

When I tell you about my trauma and drama, it is not to make myself great or to be a martyr. (Yuck!) I've spent my entire life trying to figure out how we, as humans, work. I have studied what makes us extraordinary and exceptional and why we break down. What I've discovered in the last few years is that the secret to accessing a 100% life is in perception. From perception springs the open gate leading to real potential.

So don't resist the truth. Don't wait anymore, pretending to be 100% when you are at half-mast. Be yourself. Love yourself. Breathe in and feel what you are telling yourself. Feel your truth. Raise perception to possibility. This is your path to success.

I'd like to share the formula for possibility with you. How would you like a short exercise that will position you for a 100% life? This simple exercise will unlock vitality and clarity you probably didn't even know existed inside you. You will quickly discover you can do this same process to clear the way for more love, money, health and satisfaction in your career. This process will help you to break free from virtually anything you now struggle with.

All you need is the tool to unlock the challenges in perception and I'm going to give that to you now.

Are you in?

Schedule your day with the priorities that will improve your cash flow. We so often get caught up in teaching and producing we forget about marketing. Make it a priority every day to do two important tasks related to bringing wealth in now. What your mind conceives and believes it will achieve. So make cash flow a priority and a daily habit. If you give it priority, it will give you the same due.

PERCEPTION FREEDOM FORMULA

A Simple System to Connect with Your Self-Directive and Stop Being Stuck

On my radio show, I have dedicated entire episodes to helping listeners understand the role of perception. It's a popular subject with the New Thought community, as well as with the science and the religious communities. Perception plays a huge role in our lives: we, as humans, are either greatly enhanced with great perception or are extremely held back with poor perception.

Perception defines how you will see things, how you will experience things, and how great your life can be or not be. The programs coming from the aspect of the Divine Human Blueprint called "perception" may be conscious or unconscious. Either way, these programs are affecting your ability to move forward in life. For example, let's say you are a woman who is directed to live from a perception that "a man should be the provider and take care of a woman." If you live from this program consciously or unconsciously, it will be next to impossible for you to own your own property without the help of a man. Deals will fall through, or something will happen to sabotage your success so that the program dictating this area in your perception can be validated.

I want to give you the tool that puts you in the driver's seat of life, right now!

By the way, there is a companion video that goes through the step by step process at ***http://100YouBook.com.*** I highly recommend that you watch this video, especially if you are an "immersive learner" like me.

This formula is based on something I have been teaching for years. When you combine the 100% You exercise with steps you are going to learn in this video, you will instantly unlock awareness and possibilities for yourself that you probably didn't even know were available to you. This is healthy, wealthy, loving information based on your own internal programs in perception. If your programs in perception are great, you'll be positioned for moving in the direction of your best life ever.

You can use the techniques you are about to learn to create your first breakthroughs in health, relationships, or in wealth. I am going to show you how to gain 'permission to own your life,' 'live into your life,' and 'live into your 100% possibility.' And you can do it in record time.

It's called the **"Perception Freedom Formula"** because once you have learned the technique, the door will be open for you to take charge of any and all areas of your life. Here we go:

1. Assume there are thought forms and other blocks preventing you from owning your life 100%. In perception, these could be from people who sought to dominate or control you, or group mind beliefs that are keeping you small and conforming to group standards.

   If you know how to do kinesiology (muscle testing) you can check for the number of blocks preventing you from owning your **100% life.** You'll know you're on the right track if there are 10,000 or more blocks. Everyone I read is a BIG number. I have never seen less than 7,000 impediments when muscle testing. (Reminder: this is a great time to review the video offered in this section, ***http://100YouBook.com.*** I have included an example of muscle testing and what it looks like to pump gold energy. I think you will find this video to be extremely helpful.)

2. Use your right hand, imagine pumping gold into the impediments.* Breathe deeply and be relaxed and joyous as you take charge of your life. If you have not yet discovered how to muscle test, pump gold for 10 minutes. Feel your body, breathe into your heart, and be aware of the shifts you are now feeling.
3. Next, create a list of **Frequently Experienced Problems (FEP)** that interrupt your joy, flow, experience of connection and success. For example, here were some of mine from a couple of years ago:
   - When my Internet marketing coach asked if I knew of anything that would stop me from accomplishing my goals, my response was my unpredictable health. Note that I could identify my perception as my unpredictable health in general, or I could identify the features of the problem one-by-one, i.e. citing pain, adrenal fatigue, digestive problems, etc. My way to marketing success was to first clear these thoughts about my health in perception; I began by taking 100% ownership of the issue.
   - Romantic, Divine love seemed just out of reach. My perception was that I might never meet my Divine complement (soul mate). I would then clear these thought forms and own my romantic love space.
   - There are days, and even weeks, where I am overcome with deep fatigue. The clearing I do then is to create the perception for healthy sustainable energy.

So you get the idea; look for and write down your Frequently Experienced Problems, your FEPs. Please be honest here. No one but you will see this list.

In this exercise, the goal is to become aware, not to 'fix it all' in one fell swoop. It took you lifetimes to get to where you are today; it may take you a little time to get to the bottom of everything you consider to be an issue.

Please take out your journal now and write. What are your Frequently Experienced Problems?

The other way I'd like you to look at perception and freedom is to look at **Frequent People Problems (FPP).** Frequent People Problems are problems others notice and point out to you. By the way, if you think you have no Frequent People Problems, you are likely filtering them out, or you may be thinking that these issues are of no concern to you. Think carefully and see if you can come up with at least 3 things you have heard from others that they consider to be a concern about you.

Some good examples of what you are looking for with FPPs:

From a child: *"Mom, don't interfere. You always do that and it drives me nuts."*

Check in perception for appropriate boundaries and controlling issues. (Note: if someone says to you, "you always" and "drives me nuts", in spirit, you have left a part of you either in their body or in their aura and they are feeling taken over. Helpful advice: pull your spirit back to you and they will calm down rapidly.)

"You never listen to me" or *"you are never available when I want to..."*

This may represent a narcissistic aspect in your Divine Human Blueprint program in which you are self-centered in an unhealthy way, or it could mean that their spirit has flooded your space and is now dominating your body. (If this is the case, it is time to imagine sending all of their energy that you've taken on back to them.) You can find complete directions on this process in the karma clearing meditation on my website.

"I'm worried about your...sleep habits, drinking habits, lack of exercise, sugar intake, etc."

It is helpful to clear the issue and also look at the element of addiction in perception. Frequent People Problems are often areas of your life where you have blind spots. They are the blind spots of "I don't know that I have issues here" or "I don't think I have issues here."

Yet you have most likely heard about these issues more than once, and you can keep denying culpability, or you can say, "I need to look further into this, especially if I am hearing this from another person, because, let's face it, people rarely actually tell you what they think about you. It has to be pretty big and upsetting enough to break the social code of "just leave well enough alone."

If someone is talking about something related to you that you are uncomfortable with, they are sharing the one-in-a- thousand considerations about something you do, have done, or have said that likely is not congruent with who you say you are. In other words, nine-hundred-and-ninety-nine times, folks just don't mention the issue. Be grateful and responsive when someone shares something about you that makes you feel uncomfortable about yourself. Don't say, "You're wrong," and just blow them off. Instead, look at their comment as a course correction. Say, "Okay, I'll look into that and see how I can improve." Your being willing to examine blind spots makes shifting to a higher level sooooo much easier for you.

The biggest difference between FEPs and FPPs is your awareness. FPPs will lie hidden, whereas FEPs will usually be felt in some way. FPPs dictate responses of others towards you, while FEPs direct how you understand who you are and how you *must* respond in a given situation.

Both FEPs and FFPs automatically position you in life to win or fail, to be extraordinary or mediocre, to love and be loved, or to live isolated and alone.

When your understanding of FEPs and FFPs really gets into your consciousness and you are able to fully comprehend how pervasive and impactful leaving this "trash" in perception is, you will become captivated by the processes of (1) releasing negative and unhelpful programs and (2) upgrading your existing programs with techniques such as positive daily affirmations.

For example, imagine you want to experience deeper, more fulfilling love. This is a frequent desire on the wish list of many of my clients. Now imagine that you are building a skyscraper. Unfortunately, your prime piece of land happens to be on the site of the city dump. Everywhere you turn, there are mounds of garbage piled up. Even so, your intention is to "build a skyscraper" (a better relationship), so you start to set down some supports and cement. Eventually, you create the standing structure and put four walls up. But how stable will the walls be if you build on top of a garbage heap?

You might get clever and pour cement over the garbage so you don't have to smell the rot and decay, but it's still there. Once building progresses and you proceed to the second floor of your structure, you and your engineers discover there is no real support to build multiple levels. Then you realize that your dream of building a skyscraper cannot be realized atop a mountain of garbage. Likewise, your monument to love will have no soaring heights, no breathtaking views, and no spectacular dynamics that enable you to say, "Wow! This is my dream realized!"

Yuck! Am I right? But this is exactly what you are doing if you don't clear perception and all the negative information about loving relationships that are held in your conscious or subconscious before you start in with your monument to love.

Clearing perception means removing the "garbage bags" and "debris" till the land is clear. Once the trash has been removed, you are free to excavate down as deeply as you desire. You can now set a firm foundation for your own personal "Taj Mahal of Love." The excavation you do may mean laying a new deeper foundation not only to love but also to health, wealth, or spiritual connection.

Once the trash is gone, you are free to go as deeply as you want and also to reach for the highest heights. What 99% of people have not yet realized is that you can't possibly build something of real value and real connection on top of trash, no matter how much you have spent on trainings, therapy, and investments. It's not about how committed you are. To be truly successful means you must start with a fresh, clear, well-laid foundation.

As a result, you'll quickly realize you hold the key inside your being, for the most important shifts in order to be successful and in love with your life. Clearing FEPs and FPPs is what will give you the slight advantage, as well as position you with a deep, firm foundation.

This is your journey; the answers and the challenges are unique to you. No two people are alike. All humans have attracted difficulties in perception. Clearing unneeded harmful information will propel you into the free zone for manifesting 100% YOU!

Exercise:

Here's what I want you to do. It's time to implement.

Take a moment now and write down as many FEPs and FPPs as you can in three minutes. Timing yourself while you do this will help the ideas flow through you more rapidly. It takes your "filter" off of self-editing and enables you to write more fluently.

If you write down five issues in three minutes, you'll have fifty topics for releasing in the course of only thirty minutes. Come up with as many topics as you can. You can take your time when you actually start the process of clearing and releasing. This process will create a good list for you to work from.

FEPs (Frequently Experienced Problems) FPPs (Frequent People Problems)

Once you've finished writing down your list, label them in order of importance. You are going to want to clear your most important issues first. Create a new prioritized list below using the answers in the new order you gave them from above.

Priority of importance: FEP and FPP list

A couple of notes about this process:

- First, make sure that you have watched the training video ***http://100YouBook.com***, so when you approach clearing, you will be able to pull it off properly and your results will give you the freedom you desire.
- Be willing to look a little silly and go for it. Shaking your hand, as directed, is the simplest way to do this process. It can be done from the center of your head, or from your mind, but believe me, it is a thousand times harder to do it this way, rather than to do the shaking your hand technique.

Understand this: you can't think your way out, SO SHAKE IT, BABY! And you will shake (pump) your way to freedom.

You might remember Jesus telling the parable of a rich man whose mind was consumed by his many possessions. Jesus said that it would be easier for a camel to slip through the eye of a needle than for this fella to get into heaven. We don't need camels jumping through an eye of a needle, or any impossible task to be on the forefront of our route to freedom. Using the mind to clear these issues is like the camel leaping through the eye of a sewing needle. Why work that hard when you can take the easy route?

By the way, Jesus wasn't talking about being rich in this parable; he was pointing out the attachment to worldly objects. If your focus is on possessions, and that becomes your dominating thought, you are earthbound because you are focused on "stuff." Contrary to the "stuff" mindset is the celebration of life. To be wealthy, you can "have all the stuff"—actually as much as you like—but celebrate and connect, and live life to the fullest. Keep love and celebration as your highest measure of connection and you'll do awesome with your newfound wealth (perception).

Get specific. If you find your FEPs and FPPs are vague, I encourage you to be specific. By really identifying the issue at hand, you are much more effective in your "Perception" freedom process.

Keep in mind, you are making your **first** list. You may do this process many times before you have removed all the "trash" from your Perception. Think of this as a fast track to freedom. But even if it looks like magic, the shifts and changes are rooted in scientific and spiritual principles that have been around since man's beginning. Fast is relative. To those of you who want it all NOW, this may look like a slow process. Keep in mind that your perception has been around as long as you have; for some of you, that is a very long time.

Slow and steady wins the race, in my book. Enjoy the journey and notice how things in your life continue to shift and improve. A surefire way to experience the improvements happening more frequently is to notice and be grateful for whatever shifts you are experiencing in the present moment.

Let every small shift be cause for celebration, and enjoy the journey.

If you get overly anxious about trying to produce perfection in a week or two, your experience will be a journey of frustration and disappointment. Think about it like this: it took me a lifetime, or perhaps many lifetimes, to get to where I am now. I am willing to be generous and spacious with myself around allowing the clearings to happen in perfect timing.

Now this is the cool part...

If all you got from this exercise was to take full 100% ownership of your body, and live in your body 100%, wouldn't you be light years ahead of where you were when you started? By taking full ownership and living fully in your body, you become more magnetic to what you desire. As a result, people will feel you as being more true and authentic. Can you see how your work, life, and relationships would be greatly enhanced just by accomplishing this one powerful step?

You are positioning your perception to accelerate your leadership qualities, as well as magnetizing and manifesting a great 100% life.

If you were to go even deeper and follow my simple "100% You Formula," you would have dipped into Perception and improved your essence, matter (body), energy, and fields to make you less subject to any imprint and amalgamation from others and more of the 100% you.

When you are "100% You," you'll be fully aware of what is authentically you. You will be able to live your dreams, live an energized life of focus, clarity, and momentum, and bring your blessings and your legacy into the world.

Are you understanding the power of the process yet?

Can you see how combining your clear perception, bright spirit, vibrant juicy body, enhanced energy, and realms that all support and enhance you 100% will provide you with an unimaginable life, a life of REAL fulfillment, power and wealth? Does it make sense from this space that relationships and love play out at the most connected, joyous and highest possible expression for humankind?

Can you also see how taking the time to put yourself first and foremost, getting the trash out of the way, perfecting your grounding, and building life from a deep foundation will position you as a leader? A leader others would want to follow, emulate, and receive exponential benefits from? In this scenario, you will become a true mentor. As the Law of Attraction works perfectly, you will be richly rewarded for taking the time to nurture and love yourself, for as you give to yourself, the universe will give to you.

Are you getting how opportune the time is now to take advantage of this 100% lifestyle model?

All you need, everything, in every way, is within you to be 100% YOU now.

My goal is for you to be blown away by the upside of possibility. I want to give you a taste of the incredible shifts and the powerfully authentic you that already exists within you. With the right process, the right activations and coaching, you have the ability to turn your life into your 100% life and shine brilliantly.

I can help you make this happen.

THE SECRET TO LIVING 100% ENERGIZED, FOCUSED, AND ON-TARGET EVERY DAY

How to Deeply Connect with Your 100% Divine Human Blueprint, Transform from Good to Great, and Create Your Life on Your Own Terms NOW

What I am about to share with you works for everybody, female or male, old or young. You can be an ambitious female leader, an entrepreneur, or a stay-at-home mom, a successful executive, or a fitness instructor. It doesn't matter how difficult or easy your life has been, if you have been sick or healthy, struggling with finances and cash flow, or in awesome shape or not. It doesn't matter if you were orphaned or raised by monkeys, religious, spiritual or scientific. The Divine Human Blueprint is a universal truth that has been around since the beginning of humanity. We are designed out of the Divine Human Blueprint, and you can access it now.

Why I know this will work for you is that it worked for me. Growing up, I imagined being a fairy princess bride, with lots of babies, and of course, a Prince Charming to swoop me off my feet. I imagined us dancing our way through life, just like Leslie Ann Warren in the original "Cinderella." I really thought that all my dreams were possible and were predestined to come true. In my innocence, I could not see a future of anything less than fulfilled dreams. Can you remember back to that time? Do you remember being innocent and pure, a time when you felt connected and fueled with unlimited possibility?

At 16, I got engaged, not to a prince (he was a hog farmer), and had my fairytale wedding. The babies I'd imagined started arriving when I was age nineteen. I attended church and served God and my community five days a week. I was altruistic and learned about natural, wholesome ways to raise my children. Before long, I found myself fully committed and rising in the ranks of leadership in an organization dedicated to educating new mothers about mothering and breastfeeding. At one point, I found myself leading meetings in Minnesota, Iowa and South Dakota. I sang, prayed, read scripture, and did chores, lived my life, and once in a blue moon, I would wonder *what happened to my fairy princess life?*

I knew something was wrong, but I did not know how to change my daily experience. Married to an unkind alcoholic, I went through years with no new clothes or shoes. I was a slender city girl, a hard worker for sure. I found myself pitching hog manure, hauling hogs to market, (which by the way is a very smelly, dirty job), feeding cattle with a scoop shovel out of a ten-foot high wagon, and falling "off the wagon," literally as I slipped backwards into the trough.

In the old farmhouse with its crumbling foundation, there were a plethora of dead and living mice too close to my babies. Needless to say, this early life had no fairy princess gowns, dances, or magical happenings. It was here that I experienced the death of my dream. My childhood hadn't been perfect, but I had hoped life would get better. It most certainly did not.

The death of my dreams almost killed me. By age twenty-four, I had survived my first bout of cancer. I had endured several surgeries, and I was pregnant with my third child.

It was then that with adult consciousness I began my journey of discovery. I didn't have a fancy name for that back then, but I was deep into my research as I lived through cancer. For years, illness was pervasive and permeated every aspect of my life. I experienced profound suffering, a nasty divorce, loss of my children, and becoming wheelchair bound.

The only thing back then that kept me going was my strong and deep abiding faith that I was meant for more, and that I was a cherished beloved child of God. With every cell in my body, I knew God loved me, and that I had come with a special mission.

For more than thirty years, I have studied, searched, dreamed, envisioned, survived, fought, and chanted my way to the knowledge I am sharing with you. It has been my greatest quest to discover the secrets of the Divine Human Blueprint, how we work, and what can be if everything within us is set at its full setting.

Strangely, my health, which was always my nemesis, seemed to be the vehicle from which I was learning the most. I was developing humility, awareness, and understanding as I went through treatments, pokes, prods, cutting, and medicating. Poor health, which is what eventually taught me the secrets of the Divine Human Blueprint, was the exact same issue that was keeping me from sharing what I was learning with you.

I would be strangely held back. I would experience feelings of disconnection, lose focus or momentum, or drop back into a cycle of illness, confusion and exhaustion. It was not until I tapped into the aspect of Perception in the Divine Human Blueprint that I could sustain what I had improved. This most important piece, that of perception and the effect of thousands of thought forms on my dynamic system, has been the big game changer for me in **sustainable wellness, energy, and clarity.**

Putting the Puzzle Pieces Together

My first accomplishment came a few years prior to my understanding that there actually was a Divine Human Blueprint. I regenerated my vision by praying and imagining it to be so. I had worn glasses since age eighteen, and at forty-six years of age, I decided I didn't want them anymore. My eye doctor examined my eyes after this shift, and couldn't believe the findings. He said, *"Someone must have made a mistake. Eyes do not improve at your age."* However, that was not the case. His new findings showed I no longer needed glasses.

I now have a detailed, fantastic, regeneration program for vision. In this program, the improvements are focused on not only the eyeballs themselves, but include the optic nerve and visual cortex. I believe many people want clear vision, but perception runs so strongly that they cannot have it. Clearing perception is instrumental in sustaining improvements and maintaining great eye health and vision. You'll find information on the vision program at ***http://julierenee.com/vision***.

After the success I experienced with my vision improvement, I experienced several more health and happiness disasters, though I was able to maintain clear sight. These experiences were horribly painful.

For one, I was given a date rape drug and was brutally raped. I felt like I could not survive it, but I did pull through. Shortly after that, while taking a morning stroll, I was hit by a car and landed in bed for a year, getting out only once a week in a wheelchair. It was an awful time. I was on crazy amounts of pain medication to the point where I felt like an idiot.

I have a strong will. Eventually, I decided to end the pain medications abruptly. So I "cold turkey-ed" off the meds. Over eleven days, locked in my house, I rode out the waves of panic, hallucinations, and crazy, intense bodily sensations.

This might sound like I'm exaggerating to make a point about my expertise and how low I went, so I'm going to tell you the list of medications I stopped taking that day.

My cocktail (uggh):

- Fentanyl patch (equivalent to a morphine drip)
- Up to 9 Vicodin daily

- 2500 mgs of Relafen (Ibuprofen type drug)
- Three Lorazepam—tranquilizers

For about a month from the day I started withdrawals, I cried steadily and felt intense grief and regret.

My research (what I call the period of time in which I experienced the complications and difficulties from illness, disease, and injury), took a great turn upward about seven years ago. It was then that I started to experience healthier and longer periods of time in which I felt good and also began to experience less intense downward spirals. This is when I can point to consciously starting my discovery and memory of the Divine Human Blueprint.

More things inside me grew back, including: my tonsils and adenoids, (which had been removed by the time I was three years old); my thyroid started to grow out of virtually nothing (remember that it been completely removed); and my adrenals grew back after complete failure. I was still having ups and downs, but I was now using the pieces of the Blueprint I had access to in order to stabilize and sustain the momentum of good health. These past few years have been exciting as my health moves towards 100%, and my wealth and presence in the world continue to increase by leaps and bounds.

All About YOU

Nothing is so bad you can't overcome it. Everything that is only "good" is not good enough. Think of good as a C. The devastating stuff in our lives is what we tend to want to improve first. I totally get that. But once you accomplish getting your challenges under control, then it's time to take your life from good or "fine" and rev it up to GREAT!

Your urgent problem might be an unhappy relationship, or a failure in finances that has led you to a bankruptcy or overwhelming debt. You may have very few obvious health issues. It doesn't matter. Accessing the Divine Human Blueprint will be just as important for you to understand as the person who struggles with chronic health challenges.

More Proof

Through seventeen surgeries, ten years of radiation treatments, two-and-a-half years of my life spent in a hospital bed, a year in a wheel chair, and being saddled with overwhelming medical debts twice, I learned how to rise financially to the heights of human experience. You can, too.

There is no way you can move your body and lifestyle to 100% other than by accessing the Divine Human Blueprint. It can't be done. The early Sumerians left behind information about the Divine Human Blueprint, which has somehow not seeped into our modern culture. But clues over time have been left. It is now time to remember. Wake up this sleeping giant of information within you; this is your program for greatness!

It wasn't till recently when I started clearing Perception that the improvements became permanent and my shifts towards a life at 100% started rapidly moving in the right direction.

I'd been leading workshops for five years and had written eleven manuscripts documenting and organizing all of my findings from the Blueprint. Now, with the discovery of how important perception is regarding the outcomes and results, it is time to share all. The illusive piece of perception is now firmly in place in the teachings and trainings. My plan is to move the gifts that come from the knowledge and access of the Divine Human Blueprint to you, to all your friends, and to your family.

In the past I had given this information just to the scientists, medical professionals, and healers who had a working knowledge of the healing arts. I am now finding this way to bring it to you, simply, naturally and easily. No longer will the full knowledge of the Divine Human Blueprint's complicated directions and finite details keep you from accessing it. Formerly an obscure difficult process to master, everyone who is alive can simply and naturally accomplish his or her best ever life.

Less than three years ago, I was facing another difficult issue with health, and through that challenge, I located the piece about Perception. I had at that point brought many of my glands and organs up to 100%, only to have them drop off to dangerously low levels.

Without clearing the impediments for Perception, my good work could go down the drain weeks or months after the initial restoring process. Clearing my perception was the silver bullet.

In my own health activation, I am on target, with the perfect system, and easy tools to clear away the problems that arise. When I was facing this health crisis, I was 10% healthy. My students were concerned and I was baffled. Clearing perception did the trick and my health leaped 70% in 16 short weeks! Imagine that kind of power, the power to shift, improve, restore, regenerate, manifest and love the way you imagine to experience YOU at your very, very best!

My rapid shifts up did not happen by accident. I followed a precise formula. After using this formula 130 times and replicating the same powerful shift as a result, it is no accident that the results have stuck. It's not luck. I believe you can achieve similar results if you have the right perception and a strong, passionate desire fueling the fires so you actually follow through with the actions that are necessary to live a great life.

What's this special secret ingredient? It's simple: just add the power of transformation. Human beings are by their very nature meant to transform and become greater and more than what they were. From the very beginning, the power of rising above, transforming and taking great leaps has inspired people to courage and greatness.

Think about the great athletes who overcome incredible odds to perform against the best physical specimens in the world and go on to win the Olympic gold. Or the impoverished rising up from the slums, who fulfill greatness and leadership.

There is the story of the wealthy prince, who was told he could not see God, or be enlightened, because his wealth would hold him back. All who follow the teaching of Buddha and the story of his transformation and enlightenment know the Buddha did, indeed, transform and awaken himself.

Transformation, if you think about it, is wired into everything we know and understand. Embracing your own transformation means taking the hero's journey and transforming a mediocre or ordinary life into one of greatness, mastery, vibrancy and power.

When I began this chapter, I shared my intense story of transformation from overwhelming illness and death, back to life and purpose. This story would not have been possible if I had not accessed the Divine Human Blueprint and returned to health. This story was about me and my awakening to the purpose of my life.

My story is one of purposeful struggle. Embracing the struggle caused me to go on a lifelong quest. I was searching to find the "gift" in the struggle, which ultimately was the secret to my own life and purpose.

After decades of what felt like failure, I finally found the gift.

The Divine Human Blueprint is the Missing Secret to Life Itself!

Upon learning how to access the gift, I realized the point of my life wasn't to survive in order to show the power of will and faith combined. Nor was it to change how western medicine approaches the body.

The point of my life was to **remember how to live at 100%, fully well, healthy, and in love—virtually having a life that had been unimaginable to me before.**

Once imagined, and with a path laid out to get there, I could live in my truth. As I moved into **right** living, **right** health, **right** wealth, and **right** relationship, my real mission became obvious; I am here to help other people—especially ambitious women leaders—to achieve their personal, health, and professional transformations with my programs, meditations and services.

Acknowledging this sequence is part of the secret. The system is in place to support you in attaining your transformation, no matter if it is better health you seek or a better positioning in business, freedom, a deeper love or connection, or just living in a much higher vibe. When I immersed myself fully in actualizing the Divine Human Blueprint on my behalf, heaven and earth moved for me—and it will for you, too!

Even if the concept of the Divine Human Blueprint feels "out there" to you, I encourage you to feel into the truth of this magnificent information. Scientists have studied DNA to the point that we ordinary folks think we cannot understand it because of the complexity of the information. I am not a scientist in this life, so I am amply prepared to share with you in laymen's terms how easy the Divine Human Blueprint is to access. You can make your life resonate with truth, and restore, renew, revitalize, and get unstuck in areas where you never had accomplishments or vibrant health before.

I may not know the circumstances of your life or your story, yet I do know that what would light you up and bring you a thrill is to know that you could break through any areas where you are currently stuck or on hold. Even if you have tried a hundred times before and not had the breakthrough you desired, the Divine Human Blueprint makes it possible for you to experience the transformation you seek.

The Divine Human Blueprint is the real answer to the question, *"How do I get to a 100% lifestyle?"* I encourage you to start asking yourself this question every day.

The monolithic myth is that we have no choice, and that we must get our information to manage our health, wealth, and love from the gigantic institutions. There is widespread agreement in what I referred to as "group mind" that we have no permission as individuals to "own" our authority and ground as the experts regarding our own health, wealth, and love. Those institutions are machines, churning out small bits of helpful information, and a lot of nothing else, but group mind hypnosis.

These institutions were created and set up to keep everybody statuesque. I mention this, not because I have a problem with the big institutions, but to help you see what's real and what's possible.

Have you heard about anyone in traditional science or medicine who, right now, in present time (not in theory, or some future projection), can regenerate a failed adrenal in size, function, and chemistry?

NO. The medical books say it is impossible. And yet using the Blueprint and quantum energy, I am able to help clients over and over again, get adrenals to full size, as are my apprentices. (If you have not heard of the growing issue with adrenal fatigue and failure, the adrenals shrink from plum to raisin-size when they fail. Using only the Divine Human Blueprint accessed and brought up with quantum energy, adrenals return in less than four months.)

Here again at a glance are the elements of the Divine Human Blueprint

You are made up of these elements: Perception, Essence, Matter, and Energy, and these areas are supported by Realms.

In very simple terms:

Perception
- The Word

Essence
- Spirit
- Soul
- Life Force

Matter
- Physical Body
- DNA

Energy
- Chakras and Nadis (267 mini chakras throughout the body)
- Aura
- Meridians
- Golden Rings (halo)
- Human Access Portal (entry of spirit to body, one inch above where spine meet skull)

Realms or Fields
- Origin
- Embodiment
- Quantum
- Amplification

The Divine Human Blueprint is your helper, and it serves as the mentor to your glands, organs, systems, life, career, love, and wealth when they are functioning at less than 100%.

With your life at 100% healthy, wealthy and connected, you become the sought after expert in whatever field of work you are in because you are shining brightly and resonating with truth.

You become the connection magnet, the love receptor, the money funnel. because you have, from your core, aligned your essence, which is the "you of you"—with truth. You have removed the information that is traveling with you in Perception that has nothing to do with your magnificent life. The bottom line is that you have the answer and solution inside you for all you ever dreamed of.

Your Divine Human Blueprint is the key to achieving your 100% plan and it's simple.

In my tribe, I am looking for the powerful leaders who are energetic and ambitious. These folks are awake, aware, and very importantly motivated to go deeper.

The people I am looking for are those who get it on some level and are willing to take a leap into the unknown and trust. These individuals can feel and imagine what it would be like to have their brains leap from low to 100% functionality even before it happens. They are excited to experience their brain leaping from low to 100% functionality. These are people who get it right off the bat that their lives will be profoundly better when everything in their system is working to its peak potential.

I am looking for people who search for the truth and who are willing to watch the videos, and read the articles, and listen to the audio programs that show them how it's done, and how others have experienced full transformation in their lives.

I want people to come to this process asking for irrefutable proof, because my clients actually enroll in programs and have something significant happen in their lives as a result of accessing the Divine Human Blueprint.

When you come to me and say, "Julie Renee, this area of my life is presenting an urgent, pervasive need. I refuse to live with this problem any longer. I am fully committed to shifting it for the better once and for all," with that kind of decisive commitment you are going to get incredible results.

The kind of **results** for my clients and students I am looking for include:

- Better brain, focused, clear and directed
- More sustainable natural energy, vitality and power
- Regrowth of, and fully functioning, thyroid, adrenals and other glands and organs
- Feelings of calm and serenity, an ending to panic, anxiety, and depression
- Ability to easily fuel emotional tanks
- Feeling that fun is as important as work

After the Divine Human Blueprint activations, my clients:

- Get more speaking and consulting opportunities
- Get more clients and book more sessions consistently
- Command and magnetize a better quality of prospect and client
- Typically raise their rates and speaking fees

Additionally, as perception clears, and new 100% healthy habits are activated, things that were difficult become daily habits that are easy to do. For example, if you had previously found it difficult to be out in crowds, and we cleared you in that area, you would then notice it is truly effortless to be in a crowd. As a matter of fact, you might actually enjoy it. Similarly, if you had found it distasteful to eat nutritious foods in the past, and we cleared your perception, you would enjoy healthy foods with no resistance.

In my year-long program, I require applicants to show physical, irrefutable proof that they have achieved some kind of result beyond what is considered usual or ordinary. What I am looking for are breaks with group mind that reflect the kind of results you'd get by following the status quo and the achievement of extraordinary, transformational results.

These kinds of results—the transformational results—would indicate that my students have begun accessing the Divine Human Blueprint and can repeat the process of clearing easily. When the 100% You system is understood and in place, the work of transformation becomes easy. Once you have created a "miracle" in any single area of your life, you now have a perception in your consciousness that it can be done, and you know that the result is repeatable and achievable.

The bottom line is that these people are the biggest transformers. They lead inside and out and are self-actuators.

In my business, I want to work with the believers, who waste no time, and who will implement the shifts in perception and body improvements the minute they learn how to do so. These folks are my heroes. They are the elite VIPs who fly out to my home and experience their transformation in person. You can see them on my YouTube channel and on my website. I share their stories in my books and articles because their visible wins help to create a new group mind, one where we all have full access to the Divine Human Blueprint and can readily restore, reboot, and create 100% of our dreams.

These amazing folks are the ones who are implementing the system. They are getting to 100% by accessing the Divine Human Blueprint and are using the tools daily. They are sharing their transformations with the ones they love and work with and are really moving their dreams out into the world.

I love my inner circle of VIP Program participants and Immersion students because they are leaders in a global transformation. The world is changing; my tribe is riding the wave on the crest and will have every advantage as the new era blossoms and flourishes. With a little bit of support, these leaders can become the teachers and the reachers, together connecting and creating our new reality.

The luminaries are brought into my close-knit inner circle. They spend time with me in my home, learning the secrets of the Divine Human Blueprint. Then they take their new awareness out into their communities in order to share with others and awaken them.

What we do together is extraordinary; I give my clients the Divine Human Blueprint knowledge and access points for their full use. They, like queens and kings, own, live, and blossom into the fullness of their expression.

Overcoming obstacles that cannot, according to group mind, be overcome, is my specialty. If you can see the transformation, and believe that it is possible—even if right now you don't know how it can or will be accomplished—it will happen here. So how do you get to the freedom of full access to the Divine Human Blueprint in your life, relationships, wealth spaces, and business?

Just start from where you are and improve a little every day. There are many ways that you might not be aware of to access the Divine Human Blueprint and create transformations.

To begin:

- Perform daily meditation (Meditate on a range of topics from learning related to stem cell and DNA regeneration to wealth acceleration.)
- Own your body and all parts of your body by clearing your perception. (Also, take your body to its best and strongest self through exercise and movement.)
- Clear out relationship challenges with the karma-clearing program. (You'll find this in the "Definitive Guide to Meditation Series" at ***http://JulieRenee.com/Meditation***). Then clear every person out of your field that you have ever had a connection with, whether that connection was good or bad. (This is a magical process, as love and ease become your guiding light and stress drops away.)
- Hang around the folks who are making transformations and join in their core conversations. Be inspiring and uplifting. Leave negative friends behind. Let them share with others on their wavelength, while you make a choice to up-level all of your conversations.
- Take charge. Direct the management of your 100% life by creating structures and systems you can live with and grow into that support the new you. (Find out more about meditations and programs by visiting ***http://JulieRenee.com*** and the Resources section of this book.)

I am very excited about the successful results of my clients and students who access the quantum field and the Divine Human Blueprint!

Find all our inspiring videos at ***http://JulieRenee.com/transformations.*** You will be able to view videos showing results that my clients have experienced. I guarantee that the results they report will "wow" you and support your perception that all things are possible. As you watch them, notice how each story is set with difficult challenges and how the individual is thrilled to know a new reality. Listen to the belief or faith they have, the generosity in their voice, and their palpable excitement. Imagine telling your story of transformation.

Elite One Day~ juiced and ready:

See what it feels like to experience my Elite One Day of quantum blueprint activations.

Marketing Master gets help; Launch Day saved:

Going into a big launch and feeling depleted and fuzzy, PJ Van Hulle gets a big reboot. In this video, she states she added 4,000 people rapidly to her list, and this was possible because she now had her brain back.

No More Cramps:

This doctor received a short treatment with Julie Renee at an event that left her a raving fan. The doctor was doubled over in pain and on the floor. In a matter of three minutes, she was standing and smiling. She found me in the hall a few hours later, surprised that the cramps never came back. She is now scheduled for her first one-day.

Raised from the 'Dead," a former nun's Lazarus story:

This former nun did hour-and-a-half sessions with me twice weekly for fourteen weeks. Her intestines and colon were fully regenerated. Shortly after this video, she had the colostomy bag removed and went back to living a normal life. She would now be a perfect candidate for the one-day program.

Money Breakthrough:

In this video, Steve reports that he's made more money in two weeks than he has in his entire lifetime. Money flowed easily to

Steve as he meditated his way to greater wealth. He is a student of the "Accelerate Your Wealth Program—Twenty-one Days to Your Big Wealth Breakthrough."

Adrenals Are Back!

This cancer patient, Holly, grew back her adrenal glands while fighting cancer, which surprised her. However, she had attended our year-long program and four three-day weekends; she also did daily meditations, such as the karma-clearing meditation, which she used over and over to clear all of the family and intimate connections that would interfere with her return to health.

Jill Lublin finds the Wealth Program to be effective and simple. It fits well with her busy life style and is amplifying wealth for her in wonderful ways.

Barbara Niven is so busy that she works till she drops. See how she gets real assistance.

Melissa Risdon sleeps better, feels better and has adrenals that function well.

Please take the time to check out the videos; they are important because I want you to know how these folks accomplished their transformations.

Live each day to the fullest.

FREE RESOURCES

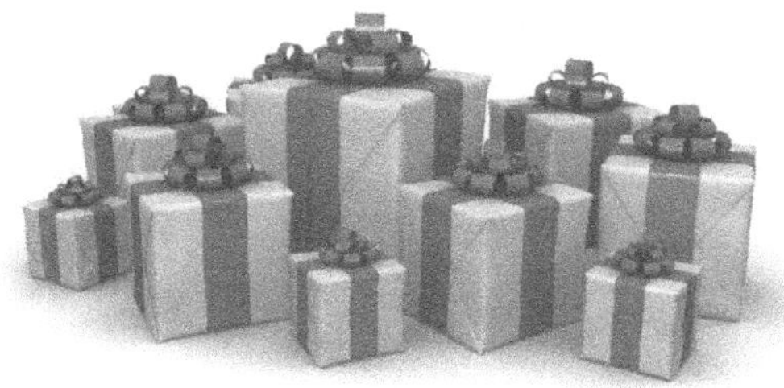

From Fatigued to Fabulous,
http://JulieRenee.com/FTF
This is a five-day program for healing adrenals and increasing good energy

Accelerate Wealth Seven-day Jumpstart,
http://JulieRenee.com/wealth

Living a Beautiful Life,
http://JulieRenee.com/beautiful
This is a Beautiful video series.

100% You Assessment on ***http://JulieRenee.com/quiz***
This assessment tells you how to find out how close you are to being 100% happy, healthy, and in love with your life.

HOW TO BEST WORK WITH YOUR DIVINE HUMAN BLUEPRINT

When I am working with you to activate your Divine Human Blueprint, we are using a **proven six-part system** that produces incredible transformation.

1. **Clear**

   The first place cleared is perception.
   We get you to:

   - 100% ownership of your body
   - 100% live in your body
   - 100% you

   After that we clear perception in the same way in your brain.

   - 100% ownership of your brain
   - 100% live in your brain
   - 100% brain

2. **Regenerate**

   Our second step is to go through each of the "five brains," getting each brain back to 100% functionality As mentioned earlier, the five brains are the instinctual, emotional, creative, logical, and genius brains.

This is the path. It's how we do the deeper work in your being using your own Divine Human Blueprint.

After several hours of improving your brain by using the Divine Human Blueprint process, your brain function goes up to 100%.

The mitochondria hold the keys to directing a cascade of new cell growth. So once the cells are fully restored, we press the program in the mitochondria that triggers a cascade of new cell growth. This process continues for ninety to one hundred and fifteen days, depending on the need. For example, if you have had a concussion at some point in your life, or traumatic brain injury, the number of days it will take for new cells to generate will be on the longer side.

Regeneration of all new brain cells creates a wondrous internal landscape for life in the body. You will experience dramatic shifts throughout your body as a result. What my clients and students notice is that all areas in the physical body begin to improve. The 100% You Divine Human Blueprint activations become permanent upgrades. In each case, perception is cleared first, then the cellular neo-genesis process becomes entirely effective. (Basically cellular neo-genesis is the growth of new cells. You can read about the complete process in my upcoming book, or in our Immersion Program course manual, which is for Immersion students only.) All shifts are created from focusing quantum energy into the area being improved.

Perception is a vital part of this transformation. When you know how to shift and remove massive negative programs and blocks, you will own the power to improve all other aspects of your life.

Shifting the brain is probably more important than you realize. In my research, I have found a brain that is clear of negative and dark influences is a brain that supports the rest of the body in moving all other aspects of health up to 100% function and chemistry.

Having your brain refreshed and your perception aligned with your 100% YOU plan can powerfully shift your wealth pictures to real wealth, not just imagined or hoped-for changes.

3. **Celebrate**
   Taking time out to acknowledge the shifts in the five brains up to 100% and the neurotransmitter function up to 100% is next. We often break here for nourishment and share a little laughter. An important part of owning your wins is acknowledging them and celebrating them, making the shift real in your conscious mind, too.

4. **Return**
   We return to the process of activation and regeneration. In this time period, we ask your being what it most wants—from calm nerves, healthy digestion, and happy hormones, to clearings in wealth, fame, or relationships. All the possible topics for human expansion, happiness and satisfaction come up here.

5. **Evaluate and Review**
   As the system of regeneration is coming to completion, it is good to revisit all of the shifts and changes that have up-leveled in the session. What are the changes you feel? What are you noticing now? Do you notice a deep state of peace? Is your mind quieter than it has ever been? Do you have a sense of well-being and a new relaxed clarity?

6. **The final step** in the system is to create your perfect steps for nurturing and follow through to support, maintain, and enhance all the upgrades you now have. You might have instructions about how and when to use meditation, or you might also have recommended shifts in diet and exercise, as well as what to do

and what not to do in the coming weeks to make your upgrades permanent and life changing.

What I have found is that regeneration and renewal are simple, natural, and easy. It is possibly the best time of your life. As the lights come on, learning becomes easier and life syncs up with your vision.

Session topics include all aspects of health, relationships, and money. What I have found is relationships of all kinds can be brought to the highest human connection by clearing harmful perceptions and then clearing each relationship. If you want to experience a new kind of relatedness, you can also do that. For example, if you always had difficulties with men, or men represented a level of pain for you, clearing thousands of programs in perception will alter your reality completely. Once the negative perceptions are cleared, you will have the capacity to feel loved and experience men as helpful, generous heroes.

Perception is what sets the magnet for what is around you, for how your body works, and even for how well your bank account and investments work. Really!

YOUR NEXT STEPS

Automate and Systematize Your Authentic Process with Full Access to the Divine Human Blueprint ~ Be 100% YOU!

What if there was a real tool that you could use to get started on your path to energy, vitality, health and having your dreams fulfilled in all areas of your life?

The 100% Healthy Divine Human Blueprint gives you access to everything.

How would you be in the world if you:

- Had permission to love yourself?
- Knew yourself as the person who is 100% healthy in the fullest definition of health?
- Felt in sync and in the flow—so that you no longer have to lead a life on autopilot where you've been settling for less than what you really want?
- Felt amazingly and joyously connected to your core essence?
- Achieved optimal health using an authentic system that is right for you?
- Experienced your whole body and being in balance?

- Were able to experience a much greater sense of spaciousness and time in your life?
- Could fuel your emotional tanks easily so that you only experienced resilience and fluidity when unexpected problems occurred?
- Felt energized and focused, could stay on track, and felt like you were being your best self?

When you experience the Divine Human Blueprint, you will notice that things you seek are moving into reach. You will feel up, and have more momentum, stamina and bounce. Wouldn't it be great to be able to exclaim: "I'm on my path to greatness!?"

Great health is important to me. I know I achieve my greatest accomplishments with great health, and I have moved my 100% healthy life to the top of my priority list.

The individualized and group courses offered along with principles in the book *100% You Formula* help your life flow. The shifts and improvements happen with grace and ease. We always begin by healing the problem areas, and then full focus can be given to creating a 100% life and lifestyle that rocks your world. Rejuvenation is more than possible; it is an expected result. Imagine having everything working as it did when you were younger-and enjoying the wisdom you have gained to get you to where you are now.

"Whatever you can do or dream you can do, believe it! Boldness has genius power and magic in it." — Goethe

CONCLUSION

Learning, without incorporating the new ways of being and implementation of those new concepts and structures, is useless. I didn't actually write this book for myself, or for the fun of it. Writing takes time and involves physical effort, time away from clients, from family, and from friends. Simply getting you pumped up with new ideas but showing no real shift was not my goal. Excitement without action leads nowhere. As I said in the introduction, living into the potential of manifesting 100% You, and the results it will generate in your life, are real and doable items. Never again will you spend useless days wishing and hoping that vitality, love, and success will find you. The book *100% You* provides the tools that, when combined with consistent and positive action, will make a real, lasting improvement in your life and lifestyle. Let this book and the new quantum tools become your guide. Let the techniques for clearing and the *100% You* success strategies sink in and produce genuine, tangible, and measurable outcomes for you.

Whenever you notice small, seemingly innocuous, "poor" thinking and behaviors not suited for your full self-expression creep back into your life, take out this book. Whenever you "fall off the wagon" of consistent self-empowerment, take out this book.

Whenever you want to reignite your "quantum" power and bolster your "why" power, take out this book. Every time you read this book, it helps to bolster your Quantum Field relationship and freedom to be more yourself.

Let me share with you what the driving force, motivations, and inspirations are for me. My core value in life is truth. My desire is to make a positive and loving difference in people's lives. So to accomplish my goal and cause a global awakening, I need *you* to experience more of your full self-expression so that you can accomplish *your* goals. It is your "testimonial of life" transformation that I'm after. I want you to receive an exciting email or letter or to have you stop me in the airport next year (or even three to five years from now) to tell me about the incredible and miraculous shifts you've realized because of the ideas you gained by reading this book. Only then will I know I have fulfilled my mission and life's purpose.

For you to get those transformational shifts (and for me to see the benefits of my testimonial), I know, from years of experience, that you have to take immediate action on your new insights and knowledge. Spiritual tools and insights left on the shelf are wasted. I don't want that to happen for you. It's time to act now on your new awarenesses and skills. You now have the power, and I expect you to own it!

You *are* ready to change your world and take charge of your dramatic improvements, right? Of course, the obvious answer is, "YES!" But you know by now that saying you're ready to make the necessary changes and actually making them isn't the same thing. To get different results, you're going to have to let go of your old ways and do things differently.

No matter where you are, or what year it is when you read this book, if I could, I'd ask you these simple questions: "Look back on your life five years ago. Are you *now*- today where you thought you would be five years later? Have you shifted up into more vitality, wealth and success? Are you in the health, love relationships, and mental clarity you wanted to be in? Do you have the cushy income, the enviable lifestyle, and the personal freedom you expected? Do you have the vibrant health, abundant loving relationships, and the world-class healing and business skills you'd intended to have by this point in your life?" If not, why? Simple: choices. It's time to make a new choice, choose to not let the next five years be a continuation of your unfulfilling past. Choose to change your life, once and for all.

Together let's make the next five years of your life miraculously better than the last five! My hope is that you've now removed your "self-delusional blinders." You know the truth about what it takes to step into living life at 100% efficiency. You've got no more excuses. Like me, you too will refuse to be fooled by the wellness latest gimmicks or become distracted by quick-fix enticements. You will stay focused on the simple, but profound, disciplines like daily meditation, exercise, and drinking enough water. These are the habits that will lead you in the direction of your dreams fulfilled. You know that nothing worth anything happens overnight. The book *100% You* exhibits the understanding that when you're committed to making moment-to-moment positive choices (despite the lack of visible or instant results), the Quantum Field *will* catapult you to heights that will astound you and inspire your friends and family. When you hold true to your "why" power and stay consistent with your new behaviors and habits, momentum will carry you swiftly forward. And then, together, with that momentum and consistent, positive action, it will be impossible for the next five years to be more of the same. On the contrary, when you put the Quantum Field to work for you, you will experience a success that, I'm willing to bet, you currently cannot imagine! It will be incredible.

I have one more valuable *100% You* activation principle to pass along to you. Whatever I want in life, I've found that the best way to get it is to focus my energy on giving it to others. If I want to boost my vitality, I look for ways to help someone else feel more vibrant and alive. If I want to feel more love cherished and inspired, I try to infuse that in someone else's day. If I want more success for myself, the fastest way to get it is to go about helping someone else feel successful.

The Field of Amplification can form a breakthrough point for good to move into the world! Think of this Field as forming a ripple effect. Imagine that you are helping others by giving generously of your time and energy to help them become more 100% themselves. You become the biggest beneficiary of your personal philanthropy. As the first simple and small step I'd like you to take in improving the trajectory of your life, I ask you to try this philosophy in your own life. If you've found value in this book, if it's helped you in any way, consider giving a copy to five people you care about and for whom you want greater success in life. The recipients could be relatives, friends, team members, or someone you just met that you would like to make a marked life difference for. I know this idea sounds as if it benefits only me. It does benefit me, along with others, but remember, I am after ever more success testimonials. My goal is to make a difference in millions of people's lives; however, to do that, I need your help. But I promise you this: Ultimately, it will be you who benefits the most. Your helping someone else find their certainty and ability to access their Quantum Field is the first step toward your exercising the *100% You* activation principles in your life. At the same time you could make a marked difference in the lives of others. Principles in this book could forever alter the courses of some people's lives, and it could be you who gives the book to them. Without you, they might not ever find these principles!

Now, write down the five people you will give a copy of this book to:

All VIP + Wealth Activation Clients

1.
2.
3.
4.
5.

Thank you for honoring me with your valuable time! I look forward to reading your *100% You* Fully Self-Expressed Success story.

~ Julie Renee

Also on JulieRenee.com

- **Free downloadable resources and worksheets** that will help you put the power of my book *100% You Formula* to work in your life. ***http://100YouBook.com***
- **Share the book *100% You Formula* with others in your life.** Special discounted pricing is available for bulk orders of the book. ***http://JulieRenee.com/BulkBooks***

More on Julie Renee

To have Julie Renee speak to your organization about the principles found in the *100% You Formula* or other Quantum Field training points, e-mail ***support@JulieRenee.com***

For more information about Julie, visit: ***www.JulieRenee.com.*** Connect with Julie and a community of like-minded, Quantum Activators online.

IT'S (FINALLY) YOUR TIME TO SHINE

So let's do this

Imagine what your life would be like if you had total 100% health, great wealth, and a career that allowed you to contribute in the most extraordinary way. With your new focus, clarity, and power, you have achieved financial freedom doing exactly what you had always dreamed you could do.

Think about how attaining your 100% status affects every element of your life. Imagine what it means for your family and your love life.

Whatever the vision is that makes you feel completely fulfilled and empowered, your 100% version of you is my commitment for you to achieve. And it is within your reach.

Get the jumpstart you may never have known was possible but has always been yours by Divine right. Begin correcting your aging and illness programs and get your vitality back. With clarity, focus, energy, and power, you can be the innovative, creative, " go-to" hero in your business, offering people ways to solve their problems (all because you've been able to solve yours and are playing with a full deck now). Start pursuing your passionate 100% life and lifestyle.

The Miracle of Water in the Body and Brain

Water gives the brain electrical energy for all brain functions, including thought and memory processes. If you experience memory lapses, drink more water. Water is vital to energy production in your cells, and in your overall metabolism, production of hormones, nerve function and neurotransmission. When your brain is functioning on full reserve of water, and you've taken in sixteen four-ounce water enhancements with the Sip Sixteen system, you will be able to think faster, be more focused, and experience greater clarity and creativity all day long.

LETS DANCE :)

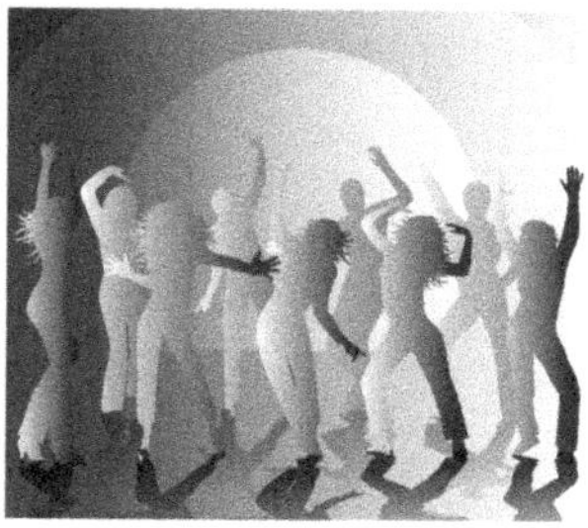

My dad used to tell us kids, "Do something or get off the pot." My dad was both a strategist and a go-getter and he lived out his dreams by going for it. He enlisted in the National Guard at the age of seventeen, served his country, came back to marry, and worked in a factory as a tool and die maker. He bought a mobile home and lost it. He and my pregnant mother then lived with his folks until he could make a course correction and buy their starter house on Quail Avenue in Crystal, Minnesota. As the years passed, they added on to the little bungalow until we were bursting at the seams, and then we moved into a four-bedroom colonial. The years have rolled on and each year my parents continue to "do something."

I have always liked this analogy: "Life is not in the candle, not in the wick or the wax, but in the burning. Live your life and live it brightly. You can choose a brighter stronger path."

There is only one way to grow back to 100% healthy, and that is through the Divine Human Blueprint. This system addresses all aspects of your life. Independence, real freedom, and financial security can be accomplished only through your Divine Human Blueprint. It's your perfect design. Every person, every woman,

man, and child has a perfect Divine Human Blueprint, a system to increase potency and true value.

If you're satisfied with living only a quarter of your true potential, then hesitate and wait. You. This system addresses all aspects down into an even weaker, less effective life. Do you want to live life with your dreams deferred indefinitely, watching others soar while you struggle and fall into the shadows?

It doesn't need to be that way. You don't need to fade into the shadows one more time, or defer your dreams another year. You can experience the 100% healthy system and learn to access your Divine Human Blueprint and incorporate it into your life. I know this is your missing piece. It is the system and process that gets you from where you are to where you want to go. Watch this video now: ***http://100YouBook.com.***

ABOUT JULIE RENEE

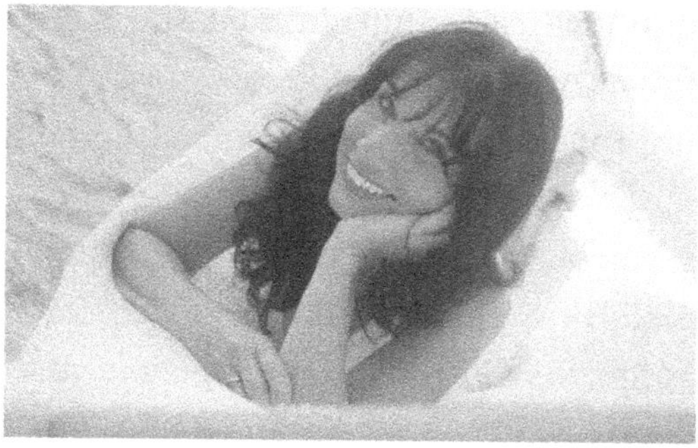

Julie Renee refuses to play small. She powerfully mentors those who are being taken out of the game with exhaustion and "fuzzy brain." She regenerates the brain and gets them back to playing at 100% again.

Books by Julie Renee are *100% You*, *Your Divine Human Blueprint*, and *Balance Your Life Now!*

Julie Renee is the founder and developer of a new spiritual science, the 100% Healthy Human Blueprint. She is the author of the groundbreaking book, Your *Divine Human Blueprint*. Her unique gift of healing defines the energy-science of Cellular Quantum Mechanics. She trains individuals in her "100% You Immersion Program" and sees private VIP clients in her home in northern California.

After launching her first business from her tiny San Francisco studio apartment in 1993, she has prevailed over a challenging history of multiple cancers and five near-death experiences. Overcoming tremendous odds, none of her doctors saw a possibility for her to survive her illnesses; she was repeatedly told she was dying. Unwilling to believe that this was true, even the Angel of Death could not convince her that it was her time to go. She has dedicated her life to the betterment of humankind and the reawakening of humanity to the Divine Human Blueprint.

Recognized for her leadership abilities, she is the recipient of the 2010-2011 National Association of Professional Women's "Woman of the Year Award" and the Powerful Women International's "Global Leadership Award" 2012.

Julie Renee has been featured as an expert on CBS, Unity FM, Rock Star Radio, Blog Talk Align, Live 365, Low Down, *Spirit Seeker, 11: 11 Magazine, Spirit Seeker Magazine,* and on various TV shows, including "New Era Healing" and a "Forum on Spirituality." She is a writer for *Holistic Fashionista Magazine* and *Accomplish Magazine*. She is also the host of the radio show, *100% Healthy*. Additionally, she has both stage and film credits, and is a harpist and singer.

Julie Renee is *the* 100% Healthy Life EXPERT. She helps women succeed in life and business by activating them simply and easily to get to 100% in both health and vitality. An expert meditation instructor, she shares the secrets of altering reality through meditation, and provides an integrated fast track for manifesting, holding and growing abundance, health, beauty, and wealth. Her home activation programs include the following:

- Beautiful From the Inside Out
- Accelerate Wealth 21 - Day Program
- Illumination Rosary for Enlightenment
- The Sound of Truth - Vedic Mantra for transformation
- Your Secret Keys audio series
- The Definitive Guide to Meditation series

- Your Divine Human Blueprint home study audio series
- Unlimited Love

As a speaker, she has shared the stage with Marci Shimoff, Jack Canfield, Caterina Rando, James Malinchak, Sean Aston, Stedman Graham, Julie Carrier, Dr. Bill Dorfman, Jill Lublin, PJ Van Hulle, and many others.

From farm wife to health activator:

Julie Renee started out in Minnesota as a farm wife, attended art school, modeled, waitressed, appeared in seven films, became a very successful realtor, and finally moved into her passion as a healer in the form of a health activator. She now has over thirty years' experience supporting individuals and groups in Quantum Health Activations, from high-risk pregnancies to life-saving interventions with critically ill individuals. Known as the premier healer for high risk pregnancies, twenty doctors and six midwives sent their most difficult clients to Julie Renee to help them from gestation through the first year after birth. In all, she has assisted more than one hundred and forty high risk babies to successfully enter this world.

Many years ago, she taught yoga and offered healing massage to people in recovery. She also taught infant massage, worked with insurance companies, and helped injured clients return to living, and hospice clients pass from this world, pain-free and without medication as they said good-by to their loved ones.

Moving deeper into her exploration of regeneration, she developed specialized Jadeite hot stone treatments, accessing the knowledge of the ancient civilizations of the Olmecs and Mayans, who used Jadeite for body initiations and transformations.

As part of a natural progression, Julie Renee moved from physical healing to offering spiritual life coaching for women. Through her clairvoyant gifts, she helped women rapidly shift to move into their next highest step.

For the past 7 years, Julie Renee has been researching and developing programs with the Blueprint, teaching through guidebooks, courses and meditation as a simple way to access the healing gifts and secrets of the Divine Human Blueprint.

Thousands of individuals have created health, wealth and love with Julie Renee's help. Through her extraordinary gifts, she has brought critically ill people back into their lives, restoring health to their cellular and energetic bodies through the Divine Human Blueprint.

Traveling the world, she has studied in India, and is both an ordained minister and a pujari (carrier of the light) in the yogic tradition.

Julie Renee's favorite vacations include rappelling down waterfalls, zip lining, and performing daring acts, such as shooting down the longest water slide in Mexico. She loves the ocean, the mountains, and nature, and is a nature girl at heart. You can find her out hiking trails every chance she gets. She challenges herself regularly by rappelling, and doing other fun but scary activities that involve hanging from great heights with ropes. Her favorite ice cream is rose petal. She loves mangos and scented flowers, especially garden roses.

Julie Renee can be reached through her website at ***www. JulieRenee.com*** or on any of the following social sites: Facebook, YouTube, LinkedIn, Twitter, and Pinterest

Who are you to play small? You who would just survive, defer dreams, and ignore gifts and talents? Having survived the worst of human health challenges, even death, itself, I ask you now if you can honestly say you are playing your life at 100%?

If the living of your life were measured like an Ivy League grading system, could you say in all aspects of your life, health, relationships, and expression that you were indeed living to your full potential? Are you planning to get your life and mission into the world in this lifetime while you have enough momentum and ability to fulfill your vision?

You were born into this life charged with a mission and a purpose. Why are you holding back? Everything you need to fulfill your divine purpose is already within you. By holding back your light, your love, your vision, you deny all of us humans the deepest gifts of your essence.

I charge you to live your life full: with a generosity and gratefulness to change heaven and earth for the betterment of all. Deny me not the privilege of your best 100% life. You are so much more then you have shared to this point. Isn't now the time to live 100%?

Inspired on the night of Nelson Mandela's passing.

YOU NEED TO KNOW

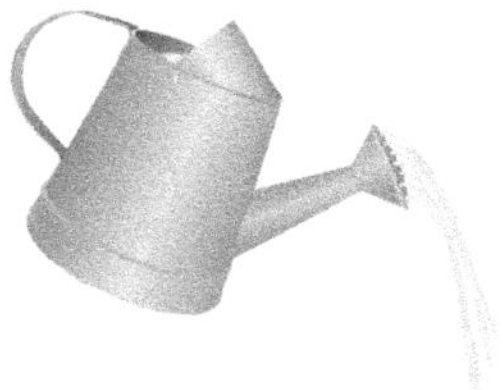

These are the things our attorney wants us to share with you.

The content case studies and examples in this book do not in any way represent the average or typical member experience. In fact, with any program offering a way to improve health, vitality, wealth, and love, we know that some members purchase our systems and never use them, and therefore, get no results from their membership at all. You should assume that you will obtain no results from this program. Therefore, the member case studies we are sharing can neither represent nor guarantee the experience of past, current, or future program participants or members. Rather, these unique case studies represent what is possible with our system. Each of these unique case studies, and any and all results reported in these case studies by individual members, are the culmination of numerous variables, many of which we cannot control, including; pre-existing mental, emotional, and health conditions, personal incentive, discontinuity of spiritual and energetic conditions, and countless other tangible and intangible factors.

When this Notice refers to "you" or "your" it means you, while "we" or "our" refers to Gable-Kennedy, Inc., dba 100% You.

Any improvements in health, mindset and energy are examples of what we think you can achieve. There are no assurances you'll do as well. If you rely only on the assurances in this book you must accept the risk of not doing as well.

Where specific health activations that have for others returned their health to high function, these examples are used and attributed to the individuals/ participants who have experienced these shifts, through 100% Healthy individual and group programs. There is no assurance you will do as well. If you rely on our 'transformations' you must also assume the risk of not doing as well.

Any representation of improved health, wealth, relationship and mindset in this book, on our websites, and in our programs are not considered to be average or normal. Likewise, any claims or representations from our course participants and students are not considered to be average results.

There can be no assurances that any prior successes, or past results, regarding health, wealth, love, and relationship can be used as an indication of future success or results.

Returning health, energy, clarity and ease to the body are based on many factors. We have no way of knowing how well you will do, as we do not know you, your background, your ability to heal, your "work" ethics or basic health and body care practices. Therefore, we do not guarantee or imply that you will have improvements or achieve better health, wealth, relationships, love, money or any other improvements suggested in this book, on our website or anywhere else. If you rely only on the assurances in this book you must accept the risk of not doing as well.

100% Healthy and 100% You programs are designed for people who are already healthy and want to take their health to the next level. Your health, wealth and love are entirely in your hands. Our programs are meant to be educational in nature and these programs may not be suited for everyone. Making decisions based on any information presented in our products, services or website should be done only with the knowledge that you could experience significant losses or make no improvements at all, or achieve no desired results regarding health, wealth, relationships, and energy.

Use caution and seek the advice of qualified professionals. Check with your health care director, therapist or professional business advisor before acting on this or any information.

Users of our products, services and website are advised to do their own due diligence when it comes to making health decisions, and all information, products and services that have been provided should be independently verified by your own qualified professional. Our information, products and services on ***www.julierenee.com*** should be carefully considered and evaluated before reaching a business decision on whether to rely on them.

You agree that our companies are not responsible for the success or failure of your health, wealth, or relationship decisions relating to the information presented on our website, ***www.julierenee.com***, or by our companies' products or services.

PRECIOUS ADVICE JUST FOR YOU FROM JULIE RENEE

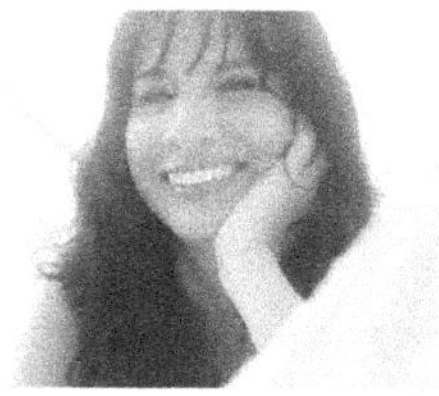

Let me help you take your next step!

You've gotten a lot of great information in this book, and hopefully a lot of value, too. If you're like me, you'll want to learn how you can take this work to the next level and get your life skyrocketing with better health, energy, connection, and momentum.

Since no two people are exactly alike, I'd like to suggest five choices about ways to take your 100% pursuit into your life. Keep in mind I have been teaching and assisting folks with health for more than two decades and am prolific. I encourage you to explore the ***www.JulieRenee.com*** website and discover a wealth of mini-programs and directed meditations if you would like to jump in with baby steps.

If, however, you like to take action in a big way and are ready to have it all, here are the three paths to choose from:

1. **100% You Assessment**
   Discover how close you are to being 100% happy healthy and in love with your life with this fun assessment and receive

instant results and helpful tools to move forward with your fully expressed 100% You life. You'll find the *100% You Formula* assessment on ***http://JulieRenee.com/quiz.***

2. **Quantum Success Activations**
   In this program, I mentor you in discovering and clearing hidden blocks to successful communication, fame, and wealth. I will teach you in a simple three-step system how to find the stops, remove them with quantum energy, and reset your success to 100%. I created this program to enhance what you have begun to master in the *100% You Formula* book found at ***http://JulieRenee.com/activate.***

3. **Julie Renee's Year of Miracle**
   We take you through the brain regeneration, which for some can start a cascade of new brain cell growth for 6 months! Now that's pretty exciting. And along with the brain we'll get a chance to work on all aspects of your being, your body will be well nurtured with rejuvenation of cells and removal of harmful DNA programs like cancer, diabetes, and even Alzheimer genes. ***http://JulieRenee.com/miracles***

I Love you and believe in your capacity to heal and be 100% YOU!

~ Julie Renee

Remember to live each day as it were your first—in awe and wonder. And live each day as if it were your last with precious awareness and appreciation because there is so much more to life than what meets the eye!